Hypnosis and Communication in Dental Practice

Hypnosis and Communication in Dental Practice

by

David Simons
Cath Potter
Graham Temple

quintessence books

Quintessence Publishing Co, Ltd
London, Berlin, Chicago, Tokyo, Barcelona, Bejing, Istanbul,
Milan, Moscow, Mumbai, Paris, Prague,
São Paulo, Seoul, and Warsaw

British Library Cataloguing in Publication Data
 Simons, David
Hypnosis and communication in dental practice
1. Hypnotism in dentistry
I. Title II. Potter, Cath III. Temple, Graham
617.6'06512

ISBN-10: 1850971161

Quintessence Publishing Co. Ltd
Grafton Road
New Malden
Surrey KT3 3AB
United Kingdom
www.quintpub.co.uk

Cover picture:
The picture shows the turbulence and calm of the River Derwent as it flows over Baslow Weir.

ISBN-10 1-85097-116-1
ISBN-13 978-1-85097-116-0

Printed in Germany

Acknowledgements

We are deeply grateful to the many practitioners and teachers who have so generously shared their knowledge with us, to the tens of thousands of patients who have given us experience in our work, and to our tireless staff, past and present, who over the years have helped to make hypnosis in dentistry such an effective and enjoyable team effort.

We also gratefully acknowledge the dedicated hard work of Mary O'Hara at Quintessence Books in bringing our work to fruition.

Preface

This book is written by dentists for dentists and the whole dental team. Whether you are a student or an experienced practitioner, you will find advice and instruction concerning vital aspects of your day-to-day interaction with patients. Excellent communication skills are an essential ingredient of patient care. When these skills are combined with hypnosis, the benefits to patients are profound. There are few disciplines where the two link together as seamlessly and as effectively as they do in dental practice.

Despite the amazing advances in dental technology and pain management that have taken place over recent years, dental treatment remains, both in folklore and in the minds of many patients, something to be feared, and it is vital that we do all we can to alleviate our patients' apprehensions. In *Hypnosis and Communication in Dental Practice* we will show you how you can reduce anxiety among your patients, and as a consequence work in a less stressful environment.

A common misconception is that hypnosis is time-consuming. On the contrary, hypnosis can save a great amount of clinical time through the use of post-hypnotic suggestions and the various other strategies that we describe. Consequently you will find that, overall, your treatment of many patients will become speedier and much more efficient.

Hypnosis is not something that you use for a particular item of treatment as you might, for example, apply a topical anaesthetic. It influences everything you do, every word you speak, every gesture you make and every facial expression you display. Hypnosis in dental practice becomes a philosophy that pervades every aspect of your own behaviour and, importantly, that of every member of your team. In *Hypnosis and Communication in Dental Practice* we demystify clinical hypnosis, demonstrating that hypnosis is not in itself a therapy but that it is a way of providing therapy by enhancing communication, thus enabling suggestions and information to be better absorbed. In this way hypnosis can be used to stimulate new ways of thinking, feeling and behaving.

The processes that we will be describing in this book begin from the first moment that a patient hears of your dental practice. That first phone call and all the interactions that take place even before you and the patient meet will have a huge impact on your relationship, and consequently upon the ease with which you and the patient can work together. Within this complex interaction the roles that the receptionist, nurses and other members of the team have to play are of paramount importance. In effect all of them will contribute to the ease with which each individual patient will accept both hypnosis and dentistry with you.

Much of this book is about the use of words. We will be examining the ways in which your choice of words, the language you use in your dental practice, has a deep influence upon the comfort and well-being of your patients. To the nervous patient every word you use carries a suggestion, and many of these words will be construed in a negative way by an anxious patient. Dentists who have learned to use hypnosis observe how their language has altered for the better, not merely in the dental practice but also in their selection and usage of words in general conversation.

In writing this book we have come to recognise the linguistic challenges of using a vocabulary that is equally applicable across genders and to all the members of the dental team, be they dental practitioners, receptionists, dental nurses, dental hygienists or dental therapists. For this reason we have generally directed our remarks in this book to you, the reader, rather than using the style of third person, "the therapist". We hope that all your team, and particularly your nursing staff, who can play such an important role in communication and hypnosis within the dental surgery, will learn from the book.

Many anxious patients are intimidated by the word "surgery", and you will read later in the book of alternative words that might be used in dental practice. However, for the sake of clarity we have chosen to use the word "surgery" within our text. We are assuming in descriptive passages, and in, for example, the sections on ideomotor signalling, induction and deepening techniques, that the dental chair and equipment are set up as for a right-handed dentist. Obviously left-handed dentists will make appropriate adjustments.

You will often find that our descriptions of the use of hypnosis will be accompanied by scripts. Initially you may want to use the scripts as written in the book as templates, but soon and inevitably your own personality and vocabulary will come into play, and we hope that quite quickly you will be using your personality and your own choice of language in your work.

The essential element of any treatment is its safety, and although hypnosis has less potential for harm than, for example, surgery, it is still possible to cause the patient considerable distress and confusion by poor technique. This book does not pretend to provide all the training required. Hypnosis is a practical subject and needs extensive practical instruction to go along with any theoretical knowledge gained. Attempting to treat conditions for which you are neither qualified nor experienced is asking for trouble.

The British Society of Medical and Dental Hypnosis provides courses in the use of hypnosis, and after sufficient training and practical experience, members can apply for Accreditation. Details for contacting both BSMDH and BSECH are given in the Appendix together with contact addresses for the RSM and Hypnosis Unit UK.

Hypnosis and Communication in Dental Practice is a team effort. The three authors come from differing backgrounds within general dental practice, hospital dentistry and dental education, and have taught hypnosis extensively to doctors, dentists and nurses. All have used hypnosis in helping patients to manage a broad range of dental concerns and medical and psychological issues.

The authors share similar views on such fundamental issues as "patient-centredness", the individuality of each patient and the importance of providing the highest quality of dental work possible. In personality and in the way these concepts are put into practice, there are inevitably, and happily, differences. That is one of the joys of working as a team.

The ultimate aim of this book is to improve the quality of your working life, and thereby to enhance the quality of dentistry for you, your patients and the entire dental team.

David Simons
Cath Potter
Graham Temple

Foreword

It is hard to escape the current debate about the emphasis on customer focus and care within the profession of dentistry. As dentists we exist for, and because of, our patients. We provide care for our patients who, if we get the product right, in turn reward us with loyalty and appreciation and the financial stability to continue to care.

Fundamental to our credibility as a profession that cares for its customers, and to overcoming barriers to that care, is the imperative for us and our dental teams to offer and provide an environment where anyone can happily, willingly and comfortably accept our advice and treatment and become a part of the community that looks after its oral health.

If we start to look carefully at the needs of the population, however, we find a huge cohort of people who don't access our services at all. There is a multitude of well-documented reasons for that, but many will certainly be anxious about attempting to start a relationship with a dentist, may be convinced that they are a "bad patient", may be scared that they just can't cope, or may simply be frightened of the fear.

The attitude of the authors of this book is that most (if not all) can benefit from hypnosis, provided that careful techniques and communication are used. Maybe by adding hypnosis and effective communication skills to our armoury of abilities we can begin to eliminate the compromises in care that are so often driven by the anxieties of our customers.

In this fascinating and encouraging book the authors have succeeded in practising what they preach. While they invite you to build rapport and relationships with your patients in a way that is accessible, appropriate, ego-strengthening and confidence-building, they have written a book pitched perfectly at a level that is accessible and at a pace that is entirely appropriate, and have developed a style that inspires confidence and an enthusiasm to use the skills you are learning.

When I was asked to write the foreword I was immediately reminded of my training in dental hypnosis many years ago with David Simons, which has so effectively coloured my own practice of dentistry, in the surgery and out of it, ever since. The skills I learned then constantly influence not only my communication with patients and colleagues but also interactions in every field of my work, and for that I am deeply grateful. Whichever way you choose to use this book – perhaps as an introduction to your own first steps in hypnosis, as a revision tool, or maybe as a means to understand the role of hypnosis in dentistry – you and your patients will certainly gain enormously from it.

Susie Sanderson
Chair, BDA Executive Board
May 2006

Contents

The History of Hypnosis in Medicine

The word "hypnosis" was coined in 1843 by a Scottish physician-surgeon James Braid who practised in Manchester. Braid carried out a great number of surgical procedures including dental extractions with hypnotised patients. He was one of the first practitioners to recognise that hypnosis was brought about by focus of attention and heightened suggestibility, and this concept became the basis of modern thinking and the teaching of hypnosis.

Prior to James Braid many explanations had been put forward to explain what we now know as hypnosis. In the past it had been thought of variously as divinely inspired, as influenced by the planets through a mysterious fluid, and as a form of magnetism. It had long been treated with suspicion, scepticism and mistrust even though its profound and beneficial effects on behaviour and on healing have been acknowledged for many centuries.

Since early history priests and witch doctors have attempted to bring about healing by inducing altered states of consciousness. In the religious and healing ceremonies of primitive peoples we see elements of the induction of a trance-like state by rhythmic drum beats and chanting, dancing and drugs, superimposed upon an elaborate ritual.

When man was searching for an explanation for the inconsistencies of life he believed disease to be a divine manifestation. Over 3,000 years ago the *Embers Papyrus*, the detailed medical text of ancient Egypt, described the Temples of Sleep where priests would give curative suggestions to patients in an induced sleep.

Asclepios and the ancients

The concept of healing within trance spread to Greece where Asclepios, revered as an inspired physician and later deified, used the phenomenon of "deep sleep", stroking the patient with his hand in order to reduce pain. Shrines and temples of healing known as Asclepieia were erected throughout Greece where the sick would come to worship and seek cures for their ills. The cult of Asclepios spread to Rome where his name became

Aesculapius, and in 293 BC a temple dedicated to him was built on an island of the Tiber where similar healing rituals took place.

Concurrently, in the British Isles the Celtic Druids were acquainted with the trance state of "Druidic sleep", which they would employ in carrying out healing.

The ancient Greek physician Hippocrates (430–377 BC), referred to now as "the father of medicine", had the inspired and innovative view that the duty of the physician was to aid nature. He taught that disease is a natural process and symptoms are the body's response to disease. He described the mind as the "seat of emotion", and concluded that the mind controlled the whole body.

Some have attributed biblical miracles and cures by holy men, relics and shrines to hypnosis, but as Christianity spread the "trance" state became regarded as a form of witchcraft and was effectively outlawed. However, Galen (AD 129–199), a Greek physician, developing the ideas of Hippocrates, proposed that the relationship between mind and body was conducted through an ethereal fluid, so emotions could influence physical health, and reciprocally physical health could influence one's mental state.

The King's Evil and medieval medicine

From the time of Edward the Confessor (1003–1066) it was assumed that that the King of England had the divine right of healing by touch. Charles II (1630–1685) is said to have healed almost 100,000 people of scrofula - tubercular swellings of the lymphatic glands in the neck. The process was approved by the Church, and a priest would always be present to read appropriate prayers as the king laid his hands on the patient.

Although the potential for healing was believed to be in the person of the king, Valentine Greatrakes, an Irish healer claiming God-given powers, also achieved many cures[1], thus long ago indicating the importance of the patient's belief system within healing.

The development of hypnosis should be seen in the context of medical science at the time. Between Roman times and the sixteenth century medicine was based largely upon religious belief, folklore, and empirical remedies with little scientific basis. Chemical anaesthesia was not introduced until the mid-nineteenth century. Prior to this alcohol and opium had been used, but surgery had been brutal and, of necessity, carried out at high speed. For example, a British surgeon, William Cheselden, is reported to have removed a stone from the bladder in 54 seconds!

Paracelsus and the universal magnetic fluid

Medical science has always been related to contemporary scientific and philosophical development. So it was in the sixteenth and seventeenth centuries, when the world's great scientists and philosophers were occupied with the relationships of the heavenly bodies and with gravity, magnetism and later, electricity, that Paracelsus (real name Theophrastus

Bombastus von Hohenheim, 1493–1541) elaborated the theory that the heavenly bodies exerted an influence upon disease and healing, working through an all-pervading universal magnetic fluid. Over the next century this theory was developed to include the concept of "animal magnetism" by which man could harness this magnetic force in order to bring about change and healing in another person.

Franz Anton Mesmer and animal magnetism

The concept of animal magnetism was to culminate in the work of Franz Anton Mesmer (1734–1815), from whom we acquired the word "mesmerism". Mesmer, a highly charismatic and ambitious physician living in Vienna, developed the theory of "animal magnetism" and he applied specially shaped magnets to the afflicted parts of patients' bodies. His success in treating an early patient for "cruel toothache and earache" led to further successes across a range of distressing conditions, and his fame, reputation and wealth increased enormously. However, in 1778 following a furore involving a young patient, Marie-Thérèse Paradis (the "blind" pianist for whom Mozart was later to write his Paradis Piano Concerto), Mesmer felt compelled to leave Vienna, moving on to Paris.

At his clinic on the rue Montmartre the patient demand was so overwhelming that he developed a form of group therapy. He set up "baquets", water baths containing magnetised iron filings from which projected iron rods that the afflicted could grip to obtain benefit from the "magnetic fluid" in the bath. Gentle music would play as Mesmer walked among the groups, wearing a lilac robe and holding an iron rod with which he would occasionally touch the patients. Many responded to this heightened atmosphere with a "convulsive crisis", and after several sessions would declare themselves cured.

In 1784 Louis XVI set up a Commission to investigate the existence of animal magnetism. The Commission concluded that the convulsive crisis that many underwent was a product of imagination and that animal magnetism did not exist[2]. Mesmer was thus discredited and moved from Paris to Spa, in Belgium. Here a group of his followers formed the Society of Harmonies, undertaking to continue the practices of Mesmer under his supervision. The Marquis de Puysegur, a member of the Society, decided that the convulsive crisis was not necessary. He believed that the magnetic power was produced in his own mind and was transferred to the patient via his fingertips. (This is the origin of hypnotic passes.)

Puysegur observed that the symptoms and behaviour of the subject could be influenced by what the "magnetiser" said. The patient would become somnambulist – a state in which they could open their eyes and talk, but remained in a magnetised sleep in which they would follow his commands. The magnetist would listen to the patient and often the patient would re-experience painful feelings. This understanding was to influence the development of talking therapies and hypnosis in ways apparent even today.

A Portuguese priest, the Abbé de Faria, practised mesmerism and wrote a seminal book in 1819 in which he rejected its basic rationale and described his concept of "lucid sleep".

De Faria introduced three radical hypotheses that relate closely to modern hypnosis: first, that approximately 20% of the populace were capable of lucid sleep, which correlates with the figures in modern studies for "highly susceptible" subjects[3]; second, that the lucid sleep facility lay within the subject rather than the mesmerist; and third, he proposed to reject the paraphernalia associated with magnetism and carry out induction simply by talking the patient into focusing their attention on "sleep".

Elliotson and Esdaile and mesmeric anaesthesia

In England John Elliotson (1791–1868) was Professor of Medicine at UCH, London. He was a larger-than-life character who made many friends but also many enemies among the medical profession. As was the custom at that time, Elliotson gave lectures and clinical demonstrations of his work to the public. His audiences included the writer Charles Dickens, who became a close friend of Elliotson, and mesmerised his own family and friends for entertainment, although he would never let himself be hypnotised.

Elliotson demonstrated a wide range of phenomena, which included profound anaesthesia while the patient was in a somnambulised state. He set up the Mesmeric Hospital in Fitzroy Square where he is reported to have carried out over 400 major operations upon somnambulised patients. Elliotson later edited a journal, *The Zoist*, in which he recorded much of his work, and importantly the work of a Scottish surgeon James Esdaile.

Esdaile (1808–1859), born in Edinburgh, obtained an appointment in the East India Company and worked as a surgeon in the Native Hospital at Hooghly in India. He carried out many hundreds of operations, apparently quite painlessly, using mesmerism as an anaesthetic. Esdaile or an assistant would produce a state akin to suspended animation, now known as the Esdaile State, by stroking the patient's body for hours over several days to "magnetise" them prior to surgery. Esdaile would then test for anaesthesia by giving the patient an electric shock or by squeezing their testicles, and only in the event of there being no response would he commence surgery.

Case history: Gooroochuan Sha, shopkeeper aged 40

> Has got a "monster tumour" [author's note: hypertrophy of the scrotum] which prevents him from moving: its great weight and his having used it as a writing desk for many years has pressed it into its present shape. His pulse is weak, his feet swollen with fluid which will make it very hazardous to attempt its removal.
>
> ... He became insensitive on the fourth day of mesmerising ... two men held the tumour in a sheet moving it forward at the same time and I removed it by a circular incision, expedition being his only safety. The rush of venous blood was great, but fortunately soon arrested ... after tying the last vessel he awoke.

The loss of blood had been so intense that he fell into a fainting state ... On recovering he said that he awoke while the mattress was being pulled back, and that nothing had disturbed him. The tumour weighed 80 lb.

I think it extremely likely that if the circulation had been hurried by pain and struggling, or if shock to the system had been increased by bodily and mental anguish, the man would have bled to death, or never have rallied from the effects of the operation. But the sudden loss of blood was all he had to contend against; and, though in so weak a condition, he has surmounted this, and gone on very well.[4]

James Esdaile reported that fatal surgical shock or post-operative infection occurred in only 5% of cases compared with the then norm of 40%. This could be explained by the elimination of stress, pain and accompanying emotional and physiological arousal that the fully conscious patient would have experienced.

When ether and chloroform came into use within Indian medical practice, Esdaile compared chemical anaesthesia unfavourably with mesmerism, claiming that the drugs had a physiologically depressive effect that could prove fatal during surgery. However, the reliability and certainty of chemical anaesthesia led to its universal adoption.

In 1846 a Boston dentist successfully anaesthetised a patient by placing an inhaler containing an ether-soaked sponge to his face, and later that same year the flamboyant London surgeon Robert Liston announced: "This Yankee dodge, gentlemen, beats mesmerism hollow"[5].

In 1852 Esdaile submitted to an English medical journal an account of 161 scrotal tumours removed during mesmeric trance. The account was rejected out of hand. An article in Lancet at that time stated:

"Mesmerism is too gross a humbug to admit of any further serious notice. We regard its abettors as quacks and impostors. They ought to be hooted out of professional Society. Any practitioner who sends a patient afflicted with any disease to consult a mesmeric quack, ought to be without clients for the rest of his days."[6]

Ill health forced Esdaile's early return from India, and he settled in Perth, Scotland, an event which was to have considerable significance.

During this same period mesmerism was being practised widely within America, much of Europe and of course within the British Isles, and there are innumerable reports of its successful use within surgery, notably as the sole anaesthetic for limb amputation, mastectomy operations and dental extractions.

An example of the scepticism professed by many luminaries of the medical profession is recorded by J. Milne Bramwell:

"In Nottinghamshire, in 1842, Mr Ward, surgeon, amputated a thigh during mesmeric trance; the patient lay perfectly calm during the whole operation, and not a muscle was seen to twitch. The case, reported to the Royal Medical and Chirurgical Society, was badly received; and it was even asserted that the patient had been trained not to express pain. Dr Marshall Hall suggested that the man was an impostor, because he had been absolutely quiet during the operation; for if he had not been simulating insensibility he should have had reflex movements in the other leg." (Topham and Ward,1842; cited in Bramwell, 1913)[7]

James Braid and hypnosis

In the mid-nineteenth century, demonstrations of mesmerism were taking place throughout the country as a form of entertainment as well as an option for treatment. In 1841 James Braid, the Manchester doctor whom we introduced at the beginning of this chapter, attended such a demonstration given by the Swiss mesmeriser M. Charles de La Fontaine. Initially Braid was extremely sceptical, but as the demonstration progressed he realised that the trance state was genuine, and decided to apply similar methods within his medical practice.

La Fontaine would normally commence by getting his subject to gaze intently, and so Braid replicated this technique by asking patients to stare at his bright lancet case and found that patients in the trance state that this seemed to produce would readily accept his suggestions aimed at cure. He believed that staring at a bright object exhausted the nervous system, bringing about a profound sleep, and that the phenomenon was not in any way related to magnetism.

In 1843 Braid published his book *Neurypnology or The Rationale of Nervous Sleep* (*neuro*: Gk nerve; and *hypnos*: Greek god of Sleep), and thus the word "hypnosis" was born.

With this revelation James Braid brought hypnosis into the realms of scientific medicine, rejecting notions of magic, magnetism or mesmerism, and asserting that the "state" could be achieved simply by concentration of the patient's attention. He carried out a broad range of surgical operations using hypnosis as the anaesthetic, but with the advent of chemical anaesthesia, hypnosis became largely redundant as an anaesthetic agent, and its practice declined in England.

Liebeault and Bernheim and suggestion theory

Not so however in France where a country physician, Dr Ambroise-August Liebeault, working predominantly with labourers and farm workers in Nancy, further developed Braid's pioneering work, placing a greater emphasis on simple suggestions of relaxation and sleep. Such was his enthusiasm and his faith in hypnosis that he would say to his patients, "If you wish me to treat you with drugs I will do so but you will have to pay me as formerly. On the other hand, if you will allow me to hypnotise you I will do it for nothing" (cited in Bramwell, 1913)[7].

Apparently Liebeault worked in an extremely low-key way, quietly giving a simple instruction to go to sleep and following this up with curative suggestions before waking the patient who might then join his friends for a chat in the doctor's waiting room before going home.

In 1882 Liebeault was joined by the initially sceptical Professor Hyppolyte Bernheim, who soon became a wholehearted supporter, and was then to work closely with him before publishing his seminal work *De la suggestion* in 1886. In this treatise Bernheim postulated that hypnosis was a special form of sleep in which suggestions were acted upon more powerfully than in the wakened state, and that hypnosis was brought about by concentrated verbal suggestion; a definition which, among many others, still holds good today.

Here a visiting professional, Franz Joseph Delboeuf, describes Bernheim's approach in hypnotising a labourer suffering from erysipelas. This was apparently the labourer's first session with Bernheim.

"Now, my friend, I am going to relieve you of all your pains; I am going to send you to sleep ... Here, I put my finger on this spot on your forehead. Do you feel the sleep coming?"
"I don't know."

"Oh! but you do. Already you can't keep your eyes open (M. Bernheim closes the man's eyes). Heaviness overwhelms all your limbs; you can't move your arm (he lifts up the patient's arm) you can't lower it. And if I make it turn (he sets it moving), you can't stop it. Even better – the more you try to stop it, the faster it will go (this happened). Let's see, where does it hurt?"
"My head."

"The pain in your head is going to go. It's away! It's gone! You have no more pain!"
"No."

" You are asleep?"
"I don't think so."

"You are asleep! You will not remember anything when you wake up. You don't feel anything (he is pricked). When you wake up you will drink half a glass of water."

"All this took scarcely the time that I need to write it. The man was deeply asleep ... He was visibly relieved of his pains [and could remember nothing of the events of the hypnosis until told to do so]."

(Delboeuf,1889; cited in Gauld, 1992)[8]

Salpêtrière: Charcot, Janet, Breuer and Freud

At this same time, at the Salpêtrière Hospital in Paris, Jean Martin Charcot, Professor of Diseases of the Nervous System, was demonstrating hypnosis on groups of female patients. Charcot still believed that magnetism was at the basis of hypnosis, and he persisted in stroking his patients with magnets. He was apparently a man of impressive intellectual power, great charisma and a colossal sense of self-worth, and at these demonstrations he asserted his view that hypnosis was a pathological state akin to hysteria, the two phenomena being interchangeable.

Following conflict between the two opposing schools of thought, Bernheim's view became accepted and Charcot's discredited. However, three of Charcot's colleagues were to have a massive impact on psychological medicine, and as the world moved into the twentieth century the emphasis within medicine, and especially within hypnosis, began to focus upon the mind, the conscious and the unconscious, and their influence upon illness, personality and behaviour.

Pierre Janet, author, philosopher and doctor of medicine, worked at Salpêtrière, collaborating with Charcot in his studies of hysteria and hypnosis. Janet developed a theory of dissociation, proposing that in hypnosis the conscious mind becomes suppressed, allowing the unconscious to surface. In deep hypnosis the unconscious mind takes control and painful memories, pushed down into the unconscious as too painful to deal with, can be exposed, often cathartically, to overcome neuroses.

Josef Breuer, a Viennese physician also working with Charcot at Salpêtrière, came to the conclusion that hysteria was caused by earlier traumatic experiences. Instead of suggesting away symptoms, he developed the application of hypnosis and changed the approach to the elimination of their apparent cause. Breuer found that in hypnosis patients would often recall past events and in talking about them would experience an emotional outpouring, subsequently losing their symptoms. He referred to this process as his "talking cure".

Sigmund Freud was born in Moravia and qualified as a physician in Vienna in 1881. Although he was principally interested in research, he was eventually to arrive at Salpêtrière to work with Charcot. In 1889 Freud went to Nancy to study hypnosis with Bernheim and Liebeault:

> *"I witnessed the moving spectacle of old Liebeault working among the poor women and children of the labouring classes. I was a spectator of Bernheim's astonishing experiments upon his hospital patients, and I received the profoundest impression of the possibility that there could be powerful mental processes which nevertheless remained hidden from the consciousness of men." (Freud 1889; cited in Gauld, 1992)*[8]

On Freud's return to Paris, he and Breuer developed a close working relationship. They used regression techniques to uncover patients' suppressed memories and named the resultant emotional outpouring "catharsis" (Gk: purging). We would now call this "abre-action". However, finding that he could not hypnotise every patient to the depth he required for his cathartic talking cure, Freud made the (in the event) momentous decision that he would give up hypnotism.

John Milne Bramwell and hypnosis in England

A huge contribution to medical hypnosis in England was made by Dr John Milne Bramwell (1852–1925), a physician practising in Wimpole Street, London. Bramwell, born in Perth, first came into contact with hypnosis as a young boy through his opportune contact with James Esdaile, who had come to live in Perth when ill health led to his leaving India. Bramwell's father was a physician, and he became a friend and colleague of Esdaile, duplicating many of his techniques in front of the boy.

In due course Bramwell qualified in medicine at Edinburgh and went into general practice, relinquishing the use of hypnosis. However, renewed enthusiasm was triggered by the events at Salpêtrière, and in 1890 he gave a demonstration in Leeds of hypnotic anaesthesia. This was reported in the *British Medical Journal* and the *Lancet*, and referrals of patients became so great that he abandoned general practice and limited himself to the practice of hypnotism.

In 1889 Bramwell had spent a fortnight in Nancy, observing Liebeault at work. Like many others before him, Bramwell was struck by the almost saintly quality of Liebeault and prophetically wrote:

> *"Though his researches have been recognized, it is certain that they have not been estimated at their true value, and that members of a younger generation have reaped the reward which his devotion of a lifetime failed to obtain."*[7]

Bramwell was frequently called in to assist dentists by inducing hypnosis in patients about to have multiple dental extractions. That he was adept in using post-hypnotic suggestions is evident from the following case report in which a young woman was referred to the Leeds dentist Arthur Turner for an extraction.

"Miss C., age 24. This patient was sent to me from another room with a note from Dr Bramwell, stating that he would not be present during the operation, and enclosing a written and signed order for her to sleep, and submit herself to my control. Upon presenting this the patient at once fell asleep.

I extracted two upper bicuspid stumps, quite buried by congested gums and very tender to the touch. I then awakened the patient, and found she was quite free from pain." (Turner, 1890; cited in Bramwell, 1913)[7]

Bramwell's book *Hypnotism, Its History, Practice and Theory*[7] remains one of the finest textbooks ever written on hypnosis in medicine.

Johannes Schultz, the Great War and autogenic training

Dr Johannes Schultz (1884-1970) studied medicine at Lausanne before specialising in psychiatry in 1909, and in 1915 he became Professor of Psychiatry at Jena.

Schultz was fascinated by the observation that patients who simply carried out verbal self-hypnosis instructions experienced a state of heaviness, well-being and warmth, and that physical concerns such as headaches and fatigue would often disappear. In 1912 this led him to write what amounted to a list of simple instructions for patients to combine with passive relaxation, and this research he published as *Autogenic Organ Exercises*.

The terrible traumas of the battlefields of the Great War resulted in 200,000 soldiers sustaining shell shock, a condition giving rise to a bizarre range of symptoms that included hysterical blindness, weird gaits and intractable shaking. On the German side, autogenic training became widely used, and for many soldiers achieved the joint aims of rapid healing from shell shock and an equally rapid return to the Front. Doctors on both sides were faced with the ethical dilemma of knowing that their role was to attempt to cure the men but also that underlying this was the need to restore the maximum number of these men to the front line as quickly as possible. In the absence of recognition of the reality of shell shock, 307 British soldiers were shot for "cowardice".

It was said that officers suffered some of the worst symptoms because they were called upon to repress their emotions to set an example for their men. Officers were treated at a number of British hospitals, of which Craiglockhart in Edinburgh was one. Here they received various drugs and electric shock treatments, rest and massage, and would have been treated by psychiatrists who, often drawing on the Freudian ideas of repressed traumas, might attempt to replicate his talking cure.

Because of the necessity for speed and the chronic shortage of drugs, hypnosis became widely used for anaesthesia during the war and increasing numbers of dentists found it invaluable as a way of minimising the trauma and pain of dental extraction, placing hypnosis in a position of respect and medical validity.

A few years after the war, Schultz moved to Berlin and in 1932 he published the first edition of *Autogenic Therapy*. The six Standard Autogenic Formulae, which form the basis of this study, shape the core of autogenic training and therapy to this day.

Between the wars: Clark Hull and Milton Erickson

Clark Hull (1884–152) came from a poor family in Akron, New York. He studied mining engineering at the University of Wisconsin, before switching to psychology, and achieved a PhD in 1918. In 1927 he studied Pavlov's research into conditioned reflexes and learning, and perceived that the work did not take account of motivational factors. He moved to the now generally discounted view that human behaviour was automatic and reducible to the language of physics, and he warned against giving subjective meanings to any of the behaviour that was being observed, although much later he was to admit this formulation probably applied only to hungry rats!

Hull was to write two major books on the subject, *Principles of Behavior* (1943) and *A Behavior System* (1952), and was to became a dominant figure in American academic psychology for 20 years.

While at Wisconsin, Hull was introduced to hypnosis, and his scientific mindset directed him towards experimentation and research, of which at that time there had been very little. It is said that as a hypnotist he regarded his subjects as inanimate laboratory objects, and therefore expected them to respond equally to induction. An important publication at this time was *Hypnosis and Suggestibility* (1933).

However, Hull's work at the University of Wisconsin was indirectly to have a colossal impact upon medical hypnosis when the young Milton Erickson attended his demonstrations and became captivated by hypnosis. Erickson quickly rejected Hull's objective, authoritarian approach, perceiving from his own experience that people responded in individual ways to induction, and could also vary in their degree of trance and the extent to which they would follow the hypnotist's suggestion. From this Erickson developed the inspiration that the therapist should enter the patient's world and let them slide into trance with whatever that patient presented at that time. He determined that when he began using hypnosis himself in his own medical practice it would be in a "naturalistic, permissive and indirect way".

It is not possible adequately to describe the life and impact of Milton Erickson (1901-1980) in this short space. Literally thousands of books and papers have been written about him and his work, and his modus operandi has been copied and distorted by a plethora of practitioners under the guise of Ericksonian techniques. He wrote with great authority on techniques of trance induction, experimental work exploring the possibilities and limits of the hypnotic experience, and investigations of the nature of the relationship between hypnotist and subject.

Erickson, brought up on a farm in Wisconsin, became doubly qualified in psychology and psychiatry. He was apparently dyslexic, tone deaf and colour-blind, being able to see only the colour purple. Like Clark Hull before him, Erickson contracted polio as a very young man, and was immobilised for many months and physically debilitated for the rest of his life. He is quoted as saying that his physical limitations had made him more observant [author's note: a valuable example of reframing], and certainly his powers of observation were legendary. For health reasons he eventually moved to Phoenix, Arizona, where he established his practice, using hypnosis throughout his career to aid clients' progression and recovery.

A major innovation in Erickson's therapeutic technique was that effective treatment was not necessarily dependent upon the formal induction of trance. He believed that his patients had problems because they were out of rapport with their unconscious minds, and that by using trance to reduce the demarcation between the conscious and unconscious minds the patient could regain rapport with his unconscious, and thus access his own resources. In addition, and crucially, his almost uncanny use of the power of language and imagery, of metaphors (often based on his own life), confusing statements, surprise and humour would cut instantaneously through to the patient's own experience and constitute a major part of his vast range of therapeutic tools.

The fact that Erickson became a cult figure would not have pleased him, any more than the fact that therapists attempting to use aspects of his technique within "Ericksonian Therapy" were often ignoring the intuitive and observational skills that the man had possessed which overrode mere technique.

Indeed there were marked parallels between Erickson and Liebeault, even though 100 years and 3,000 miles divided them. Both worked in homely, informal and non-clinical surroundings. Their personalities encompassed sharp observational powers and intuitive skills lying behind a gentleness and deep rapport and professional involvement with their patients. At the same time both men insisted on accounting for their skills in technical terms. It is also salutary to note that following them many have used their techniques, but few have achieved anything like their success.

Martin Orne: age regression and multiple personality disorder

Martin Orne was born in Vienna in 1927; his father was a surgeon and his mother a psychiatrist. The family left Austria for the USA in 1938, settling in Boston. Orne qualified as a psychologist before obtaining a medical degree and becoming a psychiatrist.

Surrounded by many sceptics, Martin Orne believed passionately in the value of hypnosis as a therapeutic tool, but even as an undergraduate at Harvard he dropped a bombshell with a paper dispelling many of the myths associated with the use of hypnosis for age regression. He proposed that the adult under hypnosis is not literally reliving his early childhood but presenting it from the perspective of adulthood. The repercussions of this were to continue to rage many years later in the controversy surrounding false memory syndrome.

A vital corollary of Orne's work was his conclusion that in crime investigation hypnosis could encourage witnesses to confabulate or "remember" things they could not actually have seen or experienced. As a result of his expertise in this field Orne was often called as an expert witness in high-profile cases, for example testifying on behalf of Patricia Hearst, the heiress who took part in a 1974 bank robbery after being held captive by the Symbionese Liberation Army.

Dr Orne also had a particular interest in the study of multiple personality disorders, and again was able to display his skills as an expert witness in a number of nationally important cases, aiding in the successful prosecution of "the Hillside Strangler", Kenneth Bianchi, convicted for ten murders and claiming a multiple personality disorder.

Ernest R. Hilgard, hypnotic susceptibility and neodissociation

Ernest Ropiequit Hilgard (1904–2001) was another giant in the development of hypnosis as a valid medical tool. He was born in Belleville, Illinois, and graduated in Chemical Engineering from the University of Illinois. He then switched to Psychology, obtaining a doctorate at Yale where he met his future wife, Josephine Rohrs, a fellow student. Hilgard became Professor of Psychology at Stanford, California in 1933. His major early interests were in learning and motivation, and two of his textbooks, *Theory of Learning* (1948) and *Introduction to Psychology* (1953), became classics.

It was in the 1950s that he and Josephine, who was by then Professor of Clinical Psychiatry at Stanford, turned their energies to hypnosis, and they became pioneers in bringing to hypnosis the discipline of scientific study, establishing the Stanford Laboratory of Hypnosis Research in 1957. Hilgard recognised a need in research for a standard by which to measure depth of hypnosis and hypnotic susceptibility, and the Stanford Hypnotic Susceptibility Scale, which he devised in 1959, is still in wide use today.

At Stanford they experimented with hypnotic pain reduction, and two books in particular, *Hypnosis in the Relief of Pain* (1975) and *Divided Consciousness* (1977), became landmarks in the objective study of hypnosis.

Hilgard further developed Janet's earlier work on dissociation into his theory of neodissociation, posing three stages of consciousness within hypnosis: the distorted reality, the hidden observer and the observing consciousness (see Chapter 2). This model, when brought together with the then contemporary Pain Gate Theory of Melzack and Wall, gave an elegant paradigm to explain the way in which hypnotic interventions can be so effective in pain management.

Post Second World War: August and Cangello

As in the Great War, shortages of analgesics and anaesthetic drugs increased the impetus for the use of hypnosis as a successful battlefield option for treatment of the injured and wounded. However, studies in peacetime indicated that hypnosis as an anaesthetic for surgery was effective in only about 10% of the population. In this context the reports in 1961 by Ralph August on 1,000 consecutive obstetric cases where hypnosis had been effective, and by Cangello on the successful management of cancer pain, served to bring hypnosis into respectability as an adjunct to mainstream medical care[9].

The call for organisation

With the advent of NHS dentistry in 1948, and the evolution of the high-speed drill, dentists were becoming more and more aware of the benefits that hypnosis could bring to their busy dental practices. The widespread fears and anxieties that so many patients brought to the surgery and the obvious continuous day-to-day necessity for analgesia focused the minds of increasing numbers of dentists upon the advantages that hypnosis could bring in reducing tensions within a stressful working environment.

As a consequence, in 1952 The British Society of Dental Hypnosis (BSDH) was formed to inform and educate dental practitioners in hypnotic techniques. In the same year the Hypnotism Act was introduced to protect the public against dangerous practices in hypnotic shows (see Chapter 5).

Three years later a medical section was added to the BSDH, and it was renamed The Dental and Medical Society for the Study of Hypnosis. In 1955 the British Medical Association formally endorsed the practice of teaching hypnosis in medical schools, approving it as a recognised form of medical practice.

Meanwhile, under similar pressures in the USA in 1958 the American Psychological Association created a specialty in hypnosis, establishing a certifying board of examiners in both clinical and experimental hypnosis. In 1959 the American Medical Association granted hypnosis "official status" as an "adjunctive tool" in medicine. As such, it completed the professional acceptance of hypnosis.

In 1968 The British Society of Medical and Dental Hypnosis (BSMDH) was established. This became a constituent society of both the European and International Societies of Hypnosis aiming "to promote the safe and responsible use of hypnosis in medicine and dentistry and to educate both our professional colleagues and the public about hypnosis and its uses".

John Hartland and ego-strengthening

John Hartland was a psychiatrist, a member of the BSMDH, and editor of the *Journal of Medical Hypnosis*. He became a significant figure in the history of hypnotherapy with the publication of an article on ego-strengthening in 1960, and his comprehensive textbook on clinical hypnotherapy, *Medical and Dental Hypnosis*, was published in 1966. An important initiative in the book is the broad use of what he called the "ego-strengthening technique". Hartland claimed that he had a 70% success rate with patients in brief hypnotherapy (fewer than 20 sessions), using ego-strengthening alone, that is, without any attention to symptom removal. We will refer to ego-strengthening extensively in this book.

The mind-body connection

As noted at the beginning of this section, hypnosis and medicine in general should be viewed within the broader spectrum of the contemporary scientific, social and philosophical picture. Modern technology has made possible progress in research into psycho-neuro-immunology (PNI), the long-sought-after connection between our thoughts and emotions, nerve pathways and the body's immune system (in effect demonstrating the actual workings of the mechanism described by Hippocrates almost 2,500 years ago). In the same vein, modern technology has opened up pathways for the study of the neurophysiological basis for hypnosis.

And now

Hypnosis is currently used more widely as a facilitator for conventional medical and dental interventions than as a cure in itself. It is used in simple relaxation techniques for nervous dental and medical patients; as a first line in acute ward admission; as an adjunct to chemical sedation and anaesthesia, as well as being an agent in its own right; as relaxation therapy in the handling of stress and related disorders; in obstetrics and antenatal care; in the management of intractable pain, cancer and terminal illness; as an adjunct to psychotherapy, and in the management of a wide range of phobic, anxiety and other medical and psychological problems.

Its application in dental practice will reduce stress upon the adult or infant patient, dentist and staff. Major uses are in the facilitation of the injection of local anaesthetic, and in helping the nervous patient to tolerate dental fillings, extractions and surgery. Hypnosis can be utilised as an adjunct to chemical sedation and anaesthesia, as well as being an agent in its own right, and as relaxation therapy in the handling of stress and related disorders. More specialised techniques can be applied to pain management and across the entire range of problems that present in the dental surgery.

2

The Nature of Hypnosis

In a clinical text book, why should you read a section on theory? Indeed why should we write one? In the context of hypnosis, is there any such thing as "theory", implying scientific basis and research?

As clinicians we are taught to practice with due regard for the "evidence base" for the techniques and treatment we provide, and psychological treatments should be no exception. In fact we *do* use many techniques and treatments that have proven effectiveness, but whose mode of action is unclear at best.

Hypnosis has been extensively studied from the early days of Louis XVI's Royal Commission's investigation of the methods of Mesmer[2] (see Chapter 1). Unfortunately, the Commission dismissed the *positive* effects of Mesmer's techniques along with his theory of animal magnetism.

Present day research and theorising recognises the central role of imagination in hypnosis, with some people able to have imaginary experiences that are indistinguishable from real events[10]. Nevertheless, the precise mechanism by which hypnosis produces its effects remains elusive.

Definitions

Definitions of hypnosis are many and varied. The British Psychological Society (BPS) used the following procedural definition[11]:

"The term 'hypnosis' denotes an interaction between one person, the 'hypnotist', and another person or people, the 'subjects'. In this interaction the hypnotist attempts to influence the subjects' perceptions, feeling, thinking and behaviour by asking them to concentrate on ideas and images that may evoke the intended effects. The verbal communications that the hypnotist uses to achieve these effects are termed 'suggestions'. Suggestions differ from everyday kinds of instructions in that they imply that a 'suc-

cessful' response is experienced by the subject as having a quality of involuntariness or effortlessness. Subjects may learn to go through the hypnotic procedures on their own, and this is termed 'self-hypnosis'." (p. 3)

The American Psychological Association (APA) recently adopted a new definition[12], but even with the care taken over this, issues with this definition have been raised[13]. Both the APA and the BPS definitions are descriptive and procedural definitions rather than explanations of the mechanism of action of hypnosis or theoretically based definitions. For this we need to look at some competing theories, and examine where the next steps in research can take us.

The "Domain of Hypnosis"

A theory or model of the process of hypnosis has to explain what has been called "the domain of hypnosis"[14], differentiating between the types of behaviour and experiences that constitute "hypnosis" and those that lie outside. This may sound simple, but in fact many properties and phenomena have been attributed to hypnosis that are now known to be incorrect. One well-known example is that of memory enhancement. It is now universally accepted that hypnosis does not increase accurate recall, and may actually encourage people to fabricate false memories both in therapy[11] and in witness reports[15].

The domain of hypnosis includes muscular movements (such as arm levitation), catalepsy (such as eyelids being unable to open), positive and negative hallucinations, amnesia, responses to post-hypnotic suggestions and distortions of the senses (such as pain control) (see Table 2.1).

Characteristic reports from good hypnotic subjects state that the performance of these tasks seems to happen automatically with no apparent effort on their part. For example, in a suggestion of arm levitation they would report that it felt as though the arm was moving "all by itself". In addition, hypnosis has traditionally been associated with an increase in suggestibility, making it easier for the subject to respond to the suggestions given by the hypnotist. However, this increase has recently been disputed, as studies show that non-hypnotic imaginative suggestibility is closely linked to hypnotic suggestibility[16].

The "altered state" debate

For many years researchers and clinicians using hypnosis assumed that when a person was hypnotised they entered a special state of consciousness fundamentally different from normal consciousness, and this they called a hypnotic trance. This concept was challenged in the 1950s and 1960s when researchers began to question whether hypnotic responding could be explained by normal social and psychological factors[17]. The debate has continued since then, although some workers believe that the two camps are not so far apart[17] and others believe that the debate is a distraction from studying real hypnotic phenomena[18].

There are those who continue to believe that the concept of the "hypnotic trance" is the essential nature of hypnotic responding although there seems to be a move away

Table 2-1 **Some hypnotic phenomena**

	Hypnotic phenomena
Alteration in voluntary muscles	Relaxation Paralysis of muscle groups Catalepsy
Alteration on involuntary muscles, organs and glands	Changes in heart rate Lowering of blood pressure, alteration of blood flow to the capillaries Variations in respiratory rate Changes in the alimentary system Alteration in salivary flow and perspiration Changes in metabolism Anatomical and biochemical changes, e.g. bleeding, blistering, modification of allergic skin responses
Alterations of the senses	Changes in visual ability, positive or negative Changes in hearing abilities Olfactory and gustatory changes Tactile changes including alteration in pain sensation Paraesthesias
Somnambulism	The subject can open their eyes, talk and obey instructions whilst remaining in hypnosis (see Puysegur, page 3)
Illusions and hallucinations	Positive and negative Sight, sound, taste, smell, touch, sensation (including pain)
Alteration of memory	Post hypnotic amnesia (rarely spontaneous) Partial amnesia during hypnosis, e.g. for a name or number Creation of false memories
Age regression	Not a literal reinstatement of the age regressed to
Time distortion	Usually under-estimating time in hypnosis

from using the term and towards using the alternative "altered state of consciousness" or ASC[19-23].

Nevertheless, for many people, when hypnosis is mentioned the concept of "trance" is what comes to mind. Heap and Aravind[24] give a definition of "trance" that they use in therapy:

> *"A waking state in which the person's attention is focused away from his or her surroundings and absorbed by inner experiences such as feelings, cognitions and imagery." (p. 25)*

According to this definition "trance" becomes similar to a number of everyday experiences such as being engrossed in a book or film, and daydreaming. Even with this pragmatic approach it is necessary to have some explanation for how and why hypnotic subjects respond as they do. The next sections will look in a little detail at the two competing explanations: one example of a "special process" or ASC account and an opposing "social psychological" explanation. This is a necessarily brief look at issues that have taken up whole books and journal issues in the past. Anyone with a special interest can find an overview in many standard textbooks of hypnosis[24-26].

Hilgard's neodissociation theory of hypnotic responding

Hilgard presents a hypothesis of how the mind works. He proposes that the mind is organised in a hierarchical way with many "cognitive control structures" monitored by a central control structure – the "executive ego". He explains that in hypnosis the hypnotist takes control of part of the control structure's executive ego and may change the hierarchical arrangement so that these become activated, but not represented consciously[14, 24].

To make this clearer, take the example of a hand levitation suggestion in hypnosis, assumed to create a "split" in consciousness resulting in the arm rising, but the subject being unaware of making the movement. This is shown diagrammatically in Figure 2.1.

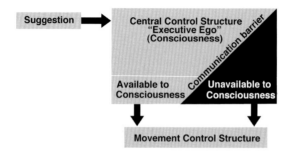

Figure 2.1 **The neodissociation account of "nonvolitional" responding**[17]

The "movement control" structure in the figure can be replaced, for example, by a "pain perception" structure or a "memory" structure.

In support of this model, highly hypnotisable individuals who, when asked if there is a part of them that is aware of the true state of affairs, for example in hypnotic pain control, report a "hidden observer" that can give a more accurate impression of the pain perceived[14, 27, 28]. This hidden observer is proposed to be the dissociated part of the "executive ego", which can be contacted, and reports levels of pain being experienced but remains hidden behind an amnesic barrier and therefore unavailable to consciousness. The hidden observer has been extensively investigated but no firm conclusions have been reached[14, 27-33].

A variation of the neodissociation theory has been proposed in which, rather than dividing the consciousness of the executive ego, hypnosis bypasses the central control structure and activates subsystems directly[34].

Further support for ASC explanations of hypnosis comes from extensive experimental research on the neurophysiology of hypnosis using EEG recordings, and newer brain imaging techniques such as fMRI and RBF[35-42]. These studies are revealing changes in the way the brain operates when hypnotisable people respond to a variety of hypnotic suggestions, including relaxation inductions and pain control sensory evoked potentials. Others believe that this does not necessarily provide evidence for an altered state of consciousness or trance and that *all* psychological processes must inevitably have neurophysiological effects[43].

Anyone who has used hypnosis will agree that some hypnotic subjects will report "trance-like experiences" during hypnosis, but the debate still remains as to whether a "hypnotic trance" is a necessary precursor to hypnosis. There is a danger of circular logic in the proposition that a "trance state" is necessary for hypnosis. The evidence for a trance state is presumed to be response to hypnotic suggestions, and the trance state is then presumed to be the *cause* of the response[24]. In addition, as has been mentioned previously, "trance-like" states are experienced in contexts outside hypnosis, and there is no way of distinguishing between causes of these other than people's self-reports of their experiences. All in all, it is probably correct to conclude that the presence of an altered state of consciousness is, as yet, unproven[44]. However, this is only half of the story, and if hypnosis is not an ASC, what is it?[18]

Sociocognitive or non-state explanations of hypnosis

There is a range of explanations that do not depend on the production of an ASC to explain hypnotic phenomena[26]. Theorists working from this perspective attempt to account for these by the normal mechanisms of human thought, behaviour and interpersonal interactions. Researchers and clinicians working from this viewpoint believe that the concept of "trance" may be a barrier to clinicians and patients alike in the effective use of hypnosis in therapy[25].

An important principle in psychology is that of Occam's razor (also referred to as the principle of parsimony), which states that when choosing between theories or models we should choose the simplest. If it is possible to explain hypnosis by ordinary psychological principles, then it is not necessary to add another concept – that of a special state or trance.

Socio-cognitive theorists vary in the weight that they give to social and cognitive factors in hypnotic responding. An early explanation was based on "Role Theory"[45]. Like Hilgard's theory, this is a theory that attempts to explain human social behaviour in general. In hypnosis the subject's expectations of how they should behave in the "role" of a hypnotic subject become emphasised. That is not to say that subjects are simply acting when they carry out suggestions, but that we all adopt roles according to our situation at any time.

The way we behave in situations is learned as part of our socialisation, and knowledge of hypnosis is widespread. This knowledge can be manipulated to affect the way people behave when they are hypnotised. An early experiment involved demonstrations of hypnosis to two groups of students by Martin Orne. In this experiment one subject exhibited spontaneous catalepsy of their dominant hand during hypnosis while the other did not. Orne commented to the group who witnessed the catalepsy demonstration that this was normal during hypnosis. When the two groups of students were hypnotised, the group who witnessed the demonstration with catalepsy tended to enact it; the other group did not[45].

Spanos[46] gives a useful overview of the types of investigations carried out to demonstrate that hypnotic responding is governed by such things as expectation, beliefs, positive attitudes and imagination. His work focuses on the types of responses that have traditionally been used as evidence that something unusual was happening in the "hypnotic state" that could not happen outside of hypnosis. An example is the claim that when good hypnotic subjects are given a suggestion that they are amnesic for something they have been told in hypnosis, it is impossible for them to remember it until the instruction is reversed. This led to the view that the forgotten material is "dissociated" from consciousness, concealed behind an amnesic barrier. However, experiments have been conducted showing that by changing the instructions, subjects *can* remember supposedly forgotten material. One experiment demonstrated that when highly hypnotisable people are told that good hypnotic subjects typically remember such things when deeply hypnotised, most of the participants did remember and correctly reported the "forgotten" items[47].

In addition, recent work has demonstrated that the main predictor of how people respond to hypnosis is how they respond to the same suggestions outside of hypnosis (so called "waking suggestion"). This has led to the proposal that hypnosis is another suggestion that people respond to like any other; in other words, the start of a hypnosis session involves the suggestion that the participant will enter a "special state" called hypnosis and the person can accept and act as if this were true[48].

Wagstaff [48] suggests that this definition allows flexibility to the description and use of hypnosis with patients: "... hypnosis can be a state of alertness, or relaxation and drowsiness; a state of focused concentration or a state of diffused attention; a state of decreased suggestibility or a state of increased suggestibility; a state of uninhibited, uncritical imaginative involvement or one of critical, analytical, convergent thought, and so on. It can be whatever is most suitable for the client" (p. 162).

This approach has obvious advantages for a clinician!

Hypnotisability

There is no disagreement among researchers that people vary in their ability to experience and respond to hypnosis. The disagreement arises in the explanations as to why this is the case. Some researchers believe that one's ability to respond to hypnosis is a fixed trait, like personality traits or IQ[14]. Evidence has been gathered to support the stability of hypnotisability scores, showing that they remain stable for twenty-five years or more[14], but it is argued that this stability could be because of the similarity in the test situation, rather than because of an innate property of the individual person[49].

It is further argued that hypnotic responsiveness can be altered by a number of methods. If a person can be convinced to expect that they will respond, they will respond to the best of their ability[49]. That is not to say that people will all respond in the same way, as people differ in their imaginative abilities and cognitive skills[16]. A second argument is that people who fail to respond to hypnosis fail because they do not interpret the suggestions in the correct way; that is, they expect things to "just happen" and do not actively participate in the process[50]. This theory led to the development of the Carlton Skills Training Program which has been shown to produce gains in hypnotic responsiveness[51-53]. The final argument is that, since people differ in many ways including how they respond to hypnosis, individually tailored approaches will mean that anyone can be "highly hypnotisable". This last theory is a mainstay of the Ericksonian approach to hypnosis.

Hypnotisability can be measured on standard scales, which usually contain a variety of suggestions ranging from "easy" suggestions such as moving hands, to more difficult suggestions such as post-hypnotic responding (from the Stanford Hypnotic Clinical Scale, SHCS[54]). There are many scales to choose from and which one is used depends on the choice of the hypnotist and the use to which the data will be put. For a review of the majority of these, see Council in Kirsch et al.[25]

Laboratory and clinical hypnosis

The attitude of the authors of this book is that most (if not all) patients can benefit from hypnosis provided careful techniques and good communication are used.

The clinical and laboratory environments are very different and people respond differently. Participants in laboratory experiments are not usually typical of the general population; they are usually students, sometimes offered incentives to take part. They have no relationship with the researcher who is hypnotising them, and in many cases the hypnosis session is delivered on tape in order to minimise "interference" from inter-personal variations.

In the clinical context the relationship built between the clinician and patient is probably the key factor in the success of hypnosis or any other psychological treatment. Some clinicians routinely test their patients before using hypnosis in their treatment, and will not use hypnosis if the patient is not responsive on formal testing. Others use scales, such as the Creative Imagination Scale (CIS)[55], which can be used with or without a "trance" induction, to see which suggestions are the most effective for the individual patient. It is then possible to tailor specific induction routines and suggestions based on the results of such tests.

One problem with using hypnotisability testing in the clinic is that a patient already low in self-esteem may interpret a low score as yet another failure. In addition, clinical research has failed to find a direct relationship between hypnotisability and treatment outcome even in research on pain control, which is said to be dependent on susceptibility to hypnosis[54]. Some laboratory studies have also disputed this[56] and a recent meta-analysis concludes that hypnotic suggestion relieves pain for most people irrespective of the type of pain and that it is not possible to draw any conclusions about the relationship to hypnotic suggestibility[57].

The clinical work that we do depends upon our ability to build rapport with patients, and their belief that we can help. We and the patient construct a hypnotic situation, by our use of language, and our mutual influence on each other's belief systems. The patient brings to the partnership their motivation to succeed, and their need to do so in order to cope with their pain or anxiety. This "real" motivation is the stepping stone to the construction of a hypnotic reality in which they can succeed, regardless of an artificial measure of their "hypnotisability".

Readers can consult many papers and books on the topics introduced in this chapter and make informed decisions on their own opinions of the nature of hypnosis. I [CP] would like to agree with Wagstaff's definition[48] as the most useful and flexible way of conceptualising clinical hypnosis, allowing us to work with patients in whichever way is best for each person as an individual, with their own beliefs and ideas that they contribute to the cooperative process known as hypnosis.

Conclusions

The debate on the nature of hypnosis is far from over and is a fascinating and interesting field of study. It also has the potential to inform other areas of the search for answers to how the mind works in general. Clinicians can usefully add to the body of knowledge already amassed on the usefulness and mechanisms of action of hypnosis, and such contributions are vital if this technique is to become fully utilised for the benefit of our patients. Clinical studies of the effectiveness of hypnosis are becoming more common, but there is still a need for more, well-controlled clinical trials in all areas, particularly in dentistry.

References

1. Buckley J. Selections from note-book of Valentine Greatrakes (1663–1679). Journal of the Waterford and South-East of Ireland Archaeological Society 1912;11, 15.
2. Franklin B, Majault, Roy L, Sallin, Bailly J-S, D'Arcet, et al. Report of the commissioners charged by the King with the examination of animal magnetism. International Journal of Clinical and Experimental Hypnosis 2002;Oct. 50(4):332–3.
3. Benham G, Smith N, Nash MR. Hypnotic susceptibility scales: are the mean scores increasing? International Journal of Clinical and Experimental Hypnosis 2002;Jan. 50(1): 5–16.
4. Esdaile J. A record of cases treated in the Mesmeric Hospital, from November 1846 to May 1847, with the reports of the Official Visitors. In: Bramwell JM, ed. Hypnosis: Its History, Practice and Theory. London: Grant Richards, 1933.
5. Cock FW. The first major operation under ether in Europe. Am J Surg (Anes Suppl) 1915;29:98–105.
6. VanPelt SJ. Hypnotism and the Power Within. London: Skeffington & Son Ltd, 1950.
7. Bramwell JM, ed. Hypnotism: Its History, Practice and Theory. London: William Rider and Son Ltd, 1913.
8. Gauld A. A History of Hypnotism. Cambridge: Cambridge University Press, 1992.
9. Cangello VW. The use of hypnotic suggestion for relief in malignant disease. International Journal of Clinical and Experimental Hypnosis 1961; 9:17–22.
10. Campbell P, McConkey KM. The Franklin Commission report, in light of past and present understanding of hypnosis. International Journal of Clinical and Experimental Hypnosis 2002; Oct. 50(4):387–96.
11. The Nature of Hypnosis. A report prepared by a working party at the request of the Professional Affairs Board of The British Psychological Society. The British Psychological Society, March 2001.
12. Green JP, Barabasz AF, Barrett D, Montgomery GH. Forging Ahead: The 2003 APA Division 30 Definition of Hypnosis. International Journal of Clinical and Experimental Hypnosis 2005; Jul. 53(3), 259–64.
13. Nash MR. The importance of being earnest when crafting definitions: science and scientism are not the same thing. International Journal of Clinical and Experimental Hypnosis 2005; Jul. 53(3): 265–80.
14. Hilgard ER. A neodissociation interpretation of hypnosis. Lynn SJ, Rhue JW, eds. Theories of Hypnosis: Current Models and Perspectives. New York: Guilford Press, 1991, pp. 83–104.
15. Wagstaff GF. Hypnosis and forensic psychology. In: Kirsch I, Capafons A, Cardena-Buelna E, Amigo S, eds. 1999. Washington DC: American Psychological Association, 1999.
16. Kirsch I, Braffman W. Correlates of hypnotizability: The first empirical study. Contemporary Hypnosis 1999;16(4): 224–230.
17. Kirsch I, Lynn SJ. Altered state of hypnosis: Changes in the theoretical landscape. Am Psychol 1995;50(10):846–58.
18. Kihlstrom JF. Is hypnosis an altered state of consciousness or what? Comment. Contemporary Hypnosis 2005;22(1):34–8.
19. Naish P. Detecting hypnotically altered states of consciousness: Comment. Contemporary Hypnosis 2005;22(1):24–30.
20. Naish PL. Hypnosis: Reinstating the state. Contemporary Hypnosis 1999; 16(3):165–9.
21. Gruzelier J. Altered states of consciousness and hypnosis in the twenty-first century: Comment. Contemporary Hypnosis 2005; 22(1):1–7.

22. Spiegel D. Multileveling the playing field: Altering our state of consciousness to understand hypnosis: Comment. Contemporary Hypnosis 2005;22(1):31–3.

23. Woody EZ, Sadler P. On the virtues of virtuosos: Comment. Contemporary Hypnosis 2005;22(1):8–13.

24. Heap M, Aravind KK. Hartland's Medical and Dental Hypnosis. 4th ed. London: Churchill Livingstone, 2002.

25. Kirsch I, Capafons A, Cardena-Buelna E, Amigo S. Clinical Hypnosis and Self-regulation: Cognitive-behavioral Perspectives. Washington DC: American Psychological Association, 1999.

26. Lynn SJ, Rhue JW. Theories of Hypnosis: Current Models and Perspectives. New York: Guilford Press, 1991.

27. Spanos NP, de Groot HP, Tiller DK, Weekes JR, Bertrand LD. Trance logic duality and hidden observer responding in hypnotic, imagination control, and simulating subjects: a social psychological analysis. J Abnorm Psychol 1985;94(4):611–23.

28. Hilgard ER. Divided consciousness and dissociation. Conscious Cogn 1992;1(1):16–31.

29. Kihlstrom JF. Dissociations and dissociation theory in hypnosis: Comment on Kirsch and Lynn (1998). Psychol Bull 1998;123(2):186–91.

30. Kirsch I, Lynn SJ. Dissociating the wheat from the chaff in theories of hypnosis: Reply to Kihlstrom (1998) and Woody and Sadler (1998). Psychol Bull 1998;123(2):198–202.

31. Kirsch I, Lynn SJ. Dissociation theories of hypnosis. Psychol Bull 1998;123(1):100–15.

32. Spanos NP, Flynn DM, Gwynn MI. Contextual demands, negative hallucinations, and hidden observer responding: three hidden observers observed. British Journal of Experimental & Clinical Hypnosis 1988;Jan. 5(1):5–10.

33. Woody E, Sadler P. On reintegrating dissociated theories: Comment on Kirsch and Lynn (1998). Psychol Bull 1998;123(2):192–7.

34. Woody EZ, Bowers KS. A frontal assault on dissociated control. In: Lynn SJ, Rhue JW, eds. Dissociation: Clinical and Theoretical Perspectives. New York: Guilford Press, 1994, pp. xvii, 477.

35. Gruzelier J. A working model of the neurophysiology of hypnosis: a review of evidence. Contemporary Hypnosis 1998;15(1):3–21.

36. Gruzelier J. Altered states of consciousness and hypnosis in the twenty-first century. Contemporary Hypnosis 2005;22(1):1–7.

37. Vaitl D, Ott U, Sammer G, Gruzelier J, Jamieson GA, Lehmann D, et al. Psychobiology of altered states of consciousness. Psychol Bull 2005;131(1):98–127.

38. Horton JE, Crawford HJ, Harrington G, Downs J. Increased anterior corpus callosum size associated positively with hypnotizability and the ability to control pain. Brain 2004;127(8):1741–7.

39. Crawford HJ, Knebel T, Vendemia JM. The nature of hypnotic analgesia: neurophysiological foundation and evidence. Contemporary Hypnosis 1998;15(1):22–33.

40. Crawford HJ, Gur RC, Skolnick B, Gur RE, et al. Effects of hypnosis on regional cerebral blood flow during ischemic pain with and without suggested hypnotic analgesia. Int J Psychophysiol 1993;15(3):181–95.

41. Gruzelier JH. Redefining hypnosis: theory, methods and integration. Contemporary Hypnosis 2000;17(2):51–70.

42. Kallio S, Revonsuo A, Hämalainen H, Markela J, Gruzelier J. Anterior brain functions and hypnosis: a test of the frontal hypothesis. International Journal of Clinical and Experimental Hypnosis 2001;49(2):95–108.

43. Wagstaff GF. On the physiological redefinition of hypnosis: a reply to Gruzelier. Contemporary Hypnosis 2000;17(4):154–162.

44. Lynn SJ, Fassler O, Knox J. Hypnosis and the altered state debate: Something more or nothing more? Comment. Contemporary Hypnosis 2005;22(1):39–45.

45. Coe WC, Sarbin TR. Role theory: Hypnosis from a dramaturgical and narrational perspective. In: Lynn SJ, Rhue JW, eds. Theories of Hypnosis: Current Models and Perspectives. New York: Guilford Press, 1991, pp. 303–23.

46. Spanos NP. A sociocognitive approach to hypnosis. In: Lynn SJ, Rhue JW, eds. Theories of Hypnosis: Current Models and Perspectives. New York: Guilford Press, 1991.

47. Silva CE, Kirsch I. Breaching hypnotic amnesia by manipulating expectancy. J Abnorm Psychol 1987;96(4):325–9.

48. Wagstaff GF. The semantics and physiology of hypnosis as an altered state: Towards a definition of hypnosis. Contemporary Hypnosis 1998:15(3):149–65.

49. Kirsch I. The social learning theory of hypnosis. In: Lynn SJ, Rhue JW, eds. Theories of Hypnosis: Current Models and Perspectives. New York: Guilford Press, 1991.

50. Spanos NP, editor. A sociocognitive approach to hypnosis. In: Lynn SJ, Rhue JW, eds. Theories of Hypnosis: Current Models and Perspectives. New York: Guilford Press, 1991.

51. Spanos NP, Warnock S, de Groot HP. Cognitive skill training, confirming sensory stimuli, and responsiveness to suggestions in subjects unselected for hypnotizability. Journal of Research in Personality 1990;24(2):133–44.

52. Spanos NP, DuBreuil SC, Gabora NJ. Four-month follow-up of skill-training-induced enhancements in hypnotizability. Contemporary Hypnosis 1991; Feb. 8(1):25–32.

53. Spanos NP, Flynn DM, Gabora NJ. The effects of cognitive skill training on the Stanford Profile Scale: Form I. Contemporary Hypnosis 1993;10(1):29–33.

54. Hilgard ER, Hilgard JR. Hypnosis in the Relief of Pain. New York: Brunner/Mazel Inc, 1994.

55. Wilson SC, Barber TX. The Creative Imagination Scale as a measure of hypnotic responsiveness: applications to experimental and clinical hypnosis. Am J Clin Hypn 1978; Apr. 20(4):235–49.

56. Spanos NP, Voorneveld PW, Gwynn MI. The mediating effects of expectation on hypnotic and nonhypnotic pain reduction. Imagination, Cognition and Personality 1986;6(3):231–45.

57. Montgomery GH, DuHamel KN, Redd WH. A meta-analysis of hypnotically induced analgesia: how effective is hypnosis? International Journal of Clinical and Experimental Hypnosis 2000; Apr. 48(2):138–53.

3

Rapport in Dental Practice

Setting the scene

Hypnosis is not just a set of techniques to be used like a new piece of equipment. If you use the philosophy of hypnosis to its fullest extent it can enhance and improve your whole working life and the lives and attitudes of the staff and patients with whom you work. The aim of this chapter is to illustrate how just a few simple changes can help you to make this huge difference.

A patient's feelings about their dentist can have a dramatic effect upon their anxiety levels, and a patient's liking for their dentist can instigate the change from feeling anxious to becoming non-anxious and comfortable. This in turn can alter the entire atmosphere of the practice, leading to secondary effects upon you and your team. A succession of relaxed patients will result in a dental practice full of smiling, relaxed staff – it is considerably easier and much less enervating to work with patients who are less tense. If the practice team is relaxed relationships between members are made easier. Happy, relaxed patients and staff produce a happy, relaxed dentist! In addition, happy patients make fewer complaints and happy relaxed patients bring in more patients.

The roles of the dental team

Rapport

Why is necessary to build rapport? A simple answer is that through rapport we develop empathy, defined as "the capacity for imaginatively sharing in another's feelings or ideas". It has long been recognised that we tend to like people whom we perceive as being like us; with whom we identify and with whom we feel comfortable. So rapport enhances communication and increases mutual trust. If every time we communicate with a patient we can help them to feel more relaxed, more respected and better understood, then the benefits are shared by both of us.

When we get on well with someone we are inevitably in rapport. And within the day to day running of a dental practice it isn't necessarily anything to do with whether or not we like the other person – of necessity some of the most important rapport-building take place with patients we don't particularly like, and anyway most people are not at their best when stressed and anxious. But within a successful dental practice every comfortable interaction with every patient is dependent on establishing this special relationship; this rapport.

And the state of mind that we call "hypnosis" is a part of a continuum of behaviour by which the anxious patient arriving at the surgery unwinds and becomes amenable to treatment.

The practice ambience

A valuable exercise is to go out into the street and then approach and enter the practice as though you were an anxious patient. In fact it would be helpful to ask your staff members to carry out the same exercise.

How does the place look from the outside? And when you enter? How does it feel? Could it do with a lick of paint? Some plants?

Are the walls plastered with posters advertising dental miracles, but possibly frightening and confusing to the already frightened and confused patient? What are the smells? The sounds? How comfortable is the lighting and the furniture? Does the place feel welcoming and are you looked after?

Later in this section we will be examining the importance of words, and the implicit threat that certain words may carry.

An example of this may be the label "Surgery" on the dreaded door. Why not replace it with a sign saying "Room 2", or even simply the name of the dentist who occupies the room?

Time spent on creating a pleasant, welcoming and calming environment will be repaid many times over in its calming effect upon the whole team and upon patients, and in the development and use of hypnosis in your dental practice.

Reception staff

Reception staff are usually the first personal contact the patient has with the practice, and this contact may be by phone or face to face. The perception of your whole practice is based on how the patient reacts to this first encounter.

If they are greeted coldly or with indifference, or if difficulties seem to be put in their way, patients may respond with anger and hostility, or even just walk away. All of us welcome kindness, personal interest and help, and we must train the team to provide this.

As an example, imagine the difference between the following two exchanges:

> "Yes, what can I do for you?"
> *"Can I see the dentist today?"*
> "Are you a registered patient here?"
> *"No."*
> "Sorry, we're booked up today. I can't give you an appointment for at least a month because we're very busy. Do you want an appointment?"
> *"No thanks, I'll try somewhere else."*
> "Suit yourself."

and:

> "Hello, welcome to our dental practice. My name's Ann. How may I help you?"
> *"Can I see the dentist today?"*
> "Have you been here before?"
> *"No."*
> "Before I can give you an appointment, you need to register with us. Are you having any problems with your teeth? "
> *"No, I just want a check-up."*
> "Because our dentists are so popular, there is a bit of a wait for appointments, but I will get you in as soon as possible. Would you like me to make you an appointment?"
> *"Yes, please."*
> "Do you have any questions for us before we fill in some forms?"

Remember that communication is not just through words – the context, our body language and our facial expression can make a huge difference to the patient's perception of the meaning of words we use. A smile is essential during face-to-face contact and you may have noticed that even during a telephone conversation one party can often tell whether the other is smiling. In addition, reception staff can be trained to recognise the signals given out when a patient is anxious, and thereby to offer appropriate reassurances and alert the clinical team before the patient is seen.

The dental nurse

You should work with the dental nurse as a close team within which there must be clear and open communication. Patients may disclose quite intimate details to the dental nurse which they may shield from you, as they perceive the nurse as being more accessible and more on their level than the "powerful" dentist. The nurse's role should be as the patients' friend, who meets and greets them and imparts essential information. In turn the nurse might also then provide information for you regarding the patient's worries and concerns.

The role of dental nurses is continually being expanded and professionalised, and this is recognised by the various hypnosis societies who will now train dental nurses to use hypnosis within their job. A hypnotically trained dental nurse can be a great asset to a practice. Two hypnotists can work together, and indeed there are some induction, deepening and therapeutic techniques designed to be administered by two people. The nurse might also take over the maintenance of the hypnosis during more challenging parts of clinical procedures, allowing you to concentrate on your clinical work. In addition, a dental nurse might carry out much of the preparation, introducing the subject of hypnosis, hypnotisability testing and the teaching of self-hypnosis, as well as simple therapy for uncomplicated cases.

The dentist

You are the team leader, responsible for the maintenance of the ethos, priorities and understanding of hypnosis of the whole team. Team members can be trained to recognise the signs of dental anxiety and to respond appropriately to distressed patients. It may be necessary to convince them of the usefulness of hypnotic techniques as they may initially have preconceptions of hypnosis that mirror those of the public. Staff meetings can be useful, but direct experience of the use of hypnosis with patients will be the best way of convincing sceptical staff. Once they are persuaded of the effectiveness of hypnosis, staff can aid its use directly in their contact with patients. Hypnotic response depends to a large extent upon the positive expectation, belief and motivation of the patient. If team members are involved in the transformation of the practice into a "hypnotic practice", they will build the positive attitudes necessary for successful hypnotic responding.

Other professions complementary to dentistry

The dental team has expanded rapidly in recent years, with hygienists and increasingly dental therapists becoming essential members. Any team member who provides clinical treatment for patients can benefit from using hypnosis. For the remainder of this book the word "dentist" will be used, but it should be understood to mean any member of the dental team.

The practice environment

Although we refer to hypnotic suggestion, it is important to be aware that powerful suggestions, both positive and negative, are being given and accepted from the patient's very first contact with a dental practice. The environment of your practice can be used to give positive and reassuring suggestions to your patients before you even meet them. Successful suggestions incorporate all sensory modalities, and when we consider our practice environment we should do the same, considering sights, sounds, smells, feelings, even tastes as well as the words we use.

Sights

Avoid the temptation to use the waiting room walls as a gallery of dental techniques. A description of the latest filling techniques and implant technology may be interesting to some but, for an anxious patient may simply exacerbate anxiety. Make the area where patients sit comfortable, relaxing and neutral, with flowers, non-clinical pictures or posters, and up-to-date magazines. If children form part of your patient base, provide visual stimulation for them at their own eye level.

The dental surgery setting is usually difficult for anxious patients to deal with. Because we work there we become so familiar with the environment that we easily become desensitised and immune to the negative concepts associated with it. Look again at your surgery through fresh eyes. Store away possibly distressing instruments and equipment and "normalise" the space as far as possible. If a patient is particularly anxious, it may be necessary to carry out the initial history-taking in a neutral room away from the dental surgery, and in the case of a dental phobic outside the dental practice entirely.

Once the patient is seated in the chair provide simple, clear explanations of what they can see, remembering that what is obvious and familiar to us is far from obvious to the patient. Obviously all staff should be trained to handle instruments away from the patient's view, and to use agreed, simple and non-threatening (but accurate!) euphemisms.

Sounds: negatives and positives

Sounds can carry potent suggestions, and for most people certain pieces of music will have the effect of anchors, powerfully rekindling the feelings of an earlier experience (see Chapter 16). On the other hand, the sound of the air rotor can take an anxious patient straight back to a previous experience at the dentist, thereby reinforcing negative emotions.

Sometimes the sound will recreate the actual sensations experienced, and patients will report feeling pain even before the bur has touched the tooth. This pain can appear just as real as pain produced by a physical stimulus and cannot be dismissed as "all in the mind'.

Carefully selected music can create a highly successful distraction within the dental surgery[1]. By providing the patient with a set of headphones and a portable radio or CD player, surgery sounds can be blocked out sufficiently to enable treatment to be carried out with comfort. Many dental practices incorporate radio music playing as background sound, but sensitively chosen music can achieve more than this.

Evidence suggests that appropriate music can have a profound effect on pain perception. Studies have shown that patients listening to music require on average 50% less sedatives or anaesthetic drugs for procedures[2], and at Charing Cross Hospital staff have found that patients who listen to classical music with local anaesthesia suffer fewer complications and recover more quickly[3].

A Boston dentist, Wallace Gardner, gave 1,000 patients a small control box that played music and natural sounds. He reported that 75% of these patients needed no other form of anaesthetic, even when having teeth extracted. Eight other Boston dentists who joined in the experiment reported similar findings[4].

Suitable background music might be used for the benefit of staff as well as for the patient. Researchers studied fifty male surgeons who listened to music when operating. It was found that they had lower blood pressure and a slower heart rate than when working without music[5].

Children

For anxious children there is evidence that audio-taped stories are a more effective distraction than watching video tapes of the same story, and it is suggested that this is due to the children's closing their eyes and making greater use of their imagination[6, 7].

Potential negative effects

Although some dentists favour a calming radio station, there can be a problem with the station's unpredictability in that the music may be disrupted by the talking of continuity personnel or by advertising jingles, or pieces of unsuitable music may intrude.

In some situations relaxing music can, by association, produce undesirable effects. Sometimes the images invoked by a particular piece of music can be distressing, for example in reminding a patient of a recent bereavement or broken relationship, or in bringing to the fore some distant memory.

Although baroque music and certain pieces by Mozart are often recommended as having specific qualities promoting relaxation and well-being, inevitably there will be patients who will find such pieces irritating and complain, "I can't stand classical music!" For such patients the music can be played at a very low volume so that they are not irritated while still getting the benefits.

A Louisiana State university study showed that hard rock or heavy metal could raise blood pressure and heart rate[6], so this type of music is not suitable for anyone who is already anxious. Music appreciation is an intensely personal phenomenon, and you should keep a wide ranging stock of music CDs in order to cater for all tastes – including your own!

Smells

The sense of smell can be a strong suggestion in its own right, and in particular can be highly evocative of memories. The linkage between a smell and memory is extremely close, and a recent study has shown that a smell is better at helping recall of a memory than other sensory cues[7]. Importantly, this "smell memory" lasts a long time. A smell occurring before a negative experience becomes linked to the experience, and this is obviously a problem in dentistry when many patients questioned about dental experiences will mention the "dentist smell'. This is usually either eugenol[8] or a combination of cleaning agents such as alcohol used for cross-infection control between patients. This linkage provides a strong negative suggestion, especially for already anxious patients. It may be helpful to explain in lay language why we use eugenol, and to couple this with mention of the old folk remedy of using oil of cloves to stop toothache. You might also suggest that the use of cloves in apple pie gives a similar smell, which is generally regarded as rather pleasant.

Although it is probably impossible to eliminate all of these odours, it may be possible to reduce the impact by using pleasant odours to swamp them. Aromatherapy candles or oils can be very helpful, and it may even be possible to choose the oils associated with relaxing properties.

The patient

Greeting

Think for a moment of your own name and what it means to you. Possibly you can recall being incorrectly or inappropriately addressed, perhaps by mispronunciation or in a way that felt unduly formal or informal. Our name is our identity. It is the first thing we learn and the first thing we tell people about ourselves. Recall how embarrassed you have felt when you have met someone to whom you have been previously introduced and realise that you have forgotten their name. Our name is also coupled with our sense of dignity and is linked to our past. Addressing someone as Jennifer when she is known to her friends as Jen may bring back memories of "That is what my mum used to call me when she was cross with me."

At your practice, do you address an elderly person as Mr Jones or Mrs Smith or by their first name? One way of handling this may be to introduce oneself: "Good morning. I'm John Evans. What would you like me to call you?" An easier way is for your receptionist to ask the patient at registration how they would like to be addressed.

Body language and congruence

Do you ever spend time "people-watching"? For instance, in a restaurant, have you noticed how easy it is to recognise how well a couple are (or are not!) getting on with one another? What are the signs that you become aware of? Maybe they are smiling, leaning towards one another, bodies relaxed as they gaze into one another's eyes. Possibly if one has their head cocked slightly to the side, the other also has their head tilted the same way. If one has their hands resting easily on the table then the other does as well. They tend to speak within similar patterns of volume and speed and cadence, and seem to match one another in countless other aspects of their posture and behaviour.

Maybe one of them is leaning forward, frowning, glaring across the table, speaking loudly and quickly, banging their fist on the table, while the other one has their head down, eyes possibly flickering from side to side, lips pursed, arms folded across chest, shoulders raised.

We translate a host of cues and come up with an interpretation that in most cases is quite accurate. We observe instantly that a person is happy, stressed, preoccupied or depressed. We take on board their breathing pattern, the set of their chin, of their shoulders, the "look in their eyes".

Watch politicians greeting one another. Sometimes it's so easy to tell that their meeting has all the makings of a disaster. You can tell even on a small television screen that the smiles are forced, the body language doesn't match the facial and spoken messages of welcome and goodwill; there isn't *congruence*.

Congruence occurs when people are demonstrating matching behaviour towards one another, and is defined as "the quality or state of agreeing or coinciding".

There is a further state of congruence that occurs whenever we speak, and this is the congruence between what we are saying and the way in which we are saying it. Do not be misled by a person's facial expression. A patient who is clinically depressed or terribly anxious may often present with the brightest smile. Similarly, it is wise to be aware of one's own facial expression and its impact upon the other person. The constant smile that we may have been taught is reassuring, friendly and disarming to the patient may in fact indicate to them that we are not sufficiently concerned and are not empathising with their feelings.

"Listening" to non-verbal communication

In our relationship and communication with an anxious dental patient we aim to create congruence in order to reduce the other person's anxiety, and to take the heat out of the situation in which they and we find ourselves. As we listen to the words they speak, we observe their facial expression and body language to determine whether there is congruence between their words and their feelings.

Communication, whether verbal or non-verbal, is a two-way street. We ourselves are giving off a vast array of signals. And it's no use our saying "but that's not really what I meant", because at some level, however subliminally and subconsciously, that other person will have formed all sorts of conclusions about us based on their own perceptions of our appearance and behaviour.

Remember, too, that an anxious person's perception of dentistry and of you will be based on their past and on family folklore as much as on their actual visit to your practice for treatment. So for that patient, however gentle, caring and compassionate you may see yourself as being, history is working against you, and you are tarred with the same brush as "Butcher Smith up the street who took out my tooth before it had a chance to go numb" twenty years previously.

Positioning

When you sit with a patient to discuss their history and potential treatment plan, your relative positions are crucial to the gaining of rapport. A simple strategy is to imagine the numbers ten and two on a clock face and seat yourself and the patient in those positions relative to one another. Everyone has a personal space with which they are comfortable. If we intrude on that space it causes discomfort, but if we are too far away we can be perceived as distant and unfriendly. Watch the patient carefully; if they lean away, you are possibly too close.

Among the advantages of this position are that you can be close to the patient without "invading their territory" and eye contact can easily be accessed or broken by either party. It is easy to observe the patient without the apparent confrontation or threat that this might impose were you sitting directly in front of them. Again, from this position you can more unobtrusively observe the patient's body language and facial expression.

It is also useful to have a wall clock positioned beyond the patient and within your direct line of vision. If the patient were to glimpse you taking a surreptitious glance at your watch while they were giving you a background to their fears, rapport could be irretrievably lost.

Your position regarding the patient in seated dentistry lends itself easily to this arrangement, with the added advantage that you have the mobility to adjust fairly subtly to other positions when appropriate.

Eye contact

The American comic W. C. Fields said "never trust a guy who gives you a firm handshake and looks you straight in the eye", and there is an element of truth in this statement. Think of your own feelings when you are being wooed by an overenthusiastic salesperson who has been taught to use this ploy. An anxious person will benefit from reassuring eye contact mirroring his own feelings, but will also value the option of being able to look away. After all, as the dentist, however you may feel about yourself, at that first meeting you will perhaps be perceived by the patient as being all-powerful, intimidating and judgemental.

Constant eye contact may come across to the patient as threatening and confusing, and as such act as an impediment rather than an aid to rapport-building. By the same token, too little eye contact may be construed as lack of interest. Only careful attention to the patient can determine the amount of eye contact they deem appropriate.

Always allow the patient to break eye contact if they so desire. The avoidance of eye contact can also tell you about the patient's feelings. They may be anxious or embarrassed about their teeth. When trust is established, eye contact will return to normal.

A further advantage of discretional eye contact is that you are able to affirm significant points of the patient's story by accentuating eye contacts at such points, possibly accompanied by slight nodding of the head and an appropriate facial expression.

Being at approximately the same eye level as the patient is polite. For example, you might stand to welcome the patient, but be seated when they are seated. It may be construed as rudeness to be seated when the patient first enters your room, although for a child a seated adult will appear less threatening. And much of the reassurance of empathic contact is lost if you stand over the patient, forcing them to look up to you.

Posture, mirroring, pacing and leading

Posture is indicative of emotional states and feelings, but is also sometimes a habitual behaviour. Observation of the patient's posture can be really valuable when combined with other factors described in this section.

Your own posture is also highly relevant, and can be used to help the patient feel at ease. You should be seated fairly upright, and leaning slightly forward. This position facilitates eye contact and indicates that you are ready to listen.

Before attempting to communicate verbally, it is important to observe the patient's own posture, facial expression and demeanour. Signs of anxiety or other emotional states can be recognised before a verbal exchange takes place. Notice any tension in the body, particularly watching the shoulders and hands. Is the patient perspiring? Do they appear annoyed or impatient? These non-verbal clues can help you to respond appropriately to the patient.

One rapid, effective and effortless way of gaining rapport with that patient is to *mirror* them. In our social life we mirror all the time and do it quite unconsciously. Although in the surgery this may initially seem contrived, in a very short time you will find that it feels natural and becomes almost unconscious. To mirror means what it says; in effect you become a mirror image of that person.

Mirroring is used to enhance your relationship with the patient. It is important not to "copy" exactly but to reflect the general nature of the other person's posture so that if he, for instance, were resting his chin in his right hand, your left hand would mirror the position. In the case of an anxious, tense patient, it is possible for you then to lead them into a more comfortable posture by changing yours slowly and waiting for them to follow.

Note that there are limitations and gradations of mirroring, and it is much more subtle than mimicking. For example, you would not mirror someone picking their nose but would quite possibly unobtrusively raise your own hand towards your own face in response to their movement. Obviously if the patient has a nervous twitch or facial mannerism you would not attempt to mirror that. The movements you make and the position you take up should be natural, subtle and even attenuated copies of those of the patient.

On the basis that rapport works in both directions, mirroring occurs instinctively as rapport develops. This leads to a second, and even more valuable aspect of mirroring, which is that having initially allowed yourself to be *led* by the patient, gradually and subtly you take the lead and the patient automatically and quite unconsciously will *follow* you. So we use mirroring to gain rapport, which is extremely valuable in itself; but what is even more beneficial for the patient is the way that mirroring transforms itself seamlessly and effortlessly for the patient, from leading into being led.

Let us say, for example, that the anxious patient's shoulders are raised and his head is lowered. Initially you may mirror this in an attenuated way, but over a short time, maybe as the patient is giving you his history, you will slowly allow your own shoulders to drop and you will slowly raise your head, and this will be mirrored by the patient. In other words you can carry out the beginnings of the relaxation process simply by movement and posture without even speaking.

The dynamic and natural sequel to mirroring is *pacing*, in which at first you will be matching the patient's pace, breathing and verbal patterns. Gradually as you become the "leader", you will slow down your own pace and allow the patient to follow you. As with mirroring, pacing should be subtle so that the patient is not consciously aware of it but responds to it at a subconscious level.

Think for a moment of the way that breathing rhythm, pace and depth is a mirror to one's feelings. When we are shocked or surprised we inadvertently make a sharp intake of breath, and as we regain composure we exhale. We speak of "letting my breath out in a sigh of relief". When tense and anxious, our breathing tends to be become light and rapid, and as we relax it becomes relatively deep and slow.

Now consider the way in which our speech is linked with our breathing pattern. We speak only during exhalation. We can't speak while we inhale (try it!). And so the speech of a tense person will often tend to be in fairly rapidly delivered, short "chunks" while that of a relaxed person may be more levelly and slowly delivered, and come in larger chunks.

Observe the patient closely but unostentatiously, all the time watching for these signs of nervousness and anxiety that you will be mirroring. Are the patient's arms folded, are their legs crossed, their shoulders set and hunched? From the "ten-to-two" position you can follow the breathing pattern by the rise and fall of the shoulders, chest and abdomen. Does the patient engage you with their eyes or are they closed or looking downwards or away from you? Is the patient frowning? Is he licking his lips – a signal of the dry mouth that accompanies anxiety and fear?

"Trying"

Have you ever *tried* to get to sleep? Or *tried* to give it up smoking? *Trying* to play a musical instrument, *trying* to kick a penalty goal, even *trying* to walk, imply difficulty and failure. And yet how many times have you said to a patient to "Just *try* to relax"? So the message here is please delete the word "try" from your lexicon. Realise that whether or not you are using hypnosis, the word "try" generally serves only to imply difficulty, culminating in failure.

You may find that initially you are *trying* to carry out mirroring, pacing and hypnosis, and certainly a great many patients will tell you that they have *tried* using hypnosis. Of course we all try when we are acquiring a new skill, but you will find that observation, mirroring and pacing will quickly become natural and will seem to take place quite unconsciously.

Relaxation

What are the advantages that *you* find in working with relaxed patients rather than tense patients?
- First, rapport-building becomes easier, as relaxation and rapport work together in an ascending spiral. If you feel relaxed in another's company rapport develops quickly, and similarly, as rapport grows, so relaxation can develop. People will often say "I feel much more comfortable when I'm relaxed."
- The patient's physiology is affected. His heart rate and blood pressure are lowered and muscle tonus is reduced. The lowered muscle tonus means, for example, that the patient can keep his mouth open for longer with comfort and less expenditure of energy.
- Because of the constant feedback between mind and body, physical relaxation results in a relaxed, unstressed mind, which in turn helps to deepen the physical relaxation.

- Relaxation leads to a reduction in judging and monitoring, so that self-suggestions aimed at pain reduction are more readily accepted with a resultant raising of the patient's pain threshold.
- How often in a tense situation have you felt that you have not expressed yourself well, and not clearly understood or remembered what the other person was trying to tell you? When we are relaxed and rapport has developed our communication becomes enhanced. Our "internal communication" – the organisation of our thoughts and our ability to express them – become facilitated. At the same time, we are better able to understand and organise the thoughts being expressed by the person communicating with us.
- Through this combination of rapport, physical comfort and enhanced communication, the patient will tend to be more cooperative and compliant, leading to a reciprocal feelings among yourself and staff, leading to increased efficiency within the practice.
- So at the end of a day working in excellent rapport with a series of relaxed, pain-free, comfortable, compliant, communicable patients, you and your staff will feel the advantage. All of you will have benefited from the stress-free atmosphere and have worked harmoniously, efficiently and profitably together, and will still be full of energy at the close of the day.

Going to the dentist

Perhaps you've bumped into one of your patients in a supermarket and been astonished at their relaxed bearing and their smiling greeting, when all your previous experience of this person was of the withdrawn, unsmiling and tense person that came to your surgery. A further complication is the nature of our professional relationship as individuals, and the patient's perception of what "going to see the dentist" means. Each of us will have a preconditioned concept of expectation from this interaction, and in this "game" that we play each will adapt to a behaviour pattern that is in compliance with his perception of the expected role he has to play.

Schemata

A "schema" is a cognitive structure that contains general knowledge about an event and serves to guide our behaviour during that event. In other words we learn what we can expect and how we can behave in different situations, and those expectations and behaviour become our schema, also sometimes referred to as our "script" or "frame".

Our schema will consequently impact on how we expect others to behave; for example, the behaviour we expect of a waiter in a restaurant is not the same as that we expect of a policeman stopping us in our car.

We have a schema leading us to expect certain forms of behaviour from our patients, and when this doesn't correlate with what actually happens we may make inferences that are not valid. For example, we may be wrong in expecting a young patient to behave in a dependent and subservient way, and an older, professional person to behave independently and self-assuredly and to cope easily with treatment.

We have self-schemata, and these will influence our perception of ourselves and of others and of how our relationships may develop. But our self-schemata may also be faulty and inaccurate, thus further distorting the relationship.

Patients have schemata too. Because the dental situation is unusual and differs greatly from most experiences, the patient's expectations may be sadly misjudged. For example, when else would he expect to lie supine and defenceless, at the mercy of relative strangers? Although the patient gives us permission to touch, it is important that we do so appropriately and sensitively and that we understand that the patient may be stressed or anxious during the experience.

Stress and fear can greatly influence a person's behaviour, for example in some cases promoting an air of bravado and in others a state of withdrawal.

The patient's and our own expectations will have a significant impact upon the nature of both our personal and our professional relationships.

The transactional analysis model

The originator of transactional analysis (TA), Eric Berne[9], asserted that an individual normally exhibits three *primary ego states*, namely the Parent, the Child and the Adult, and although these ego states may overlap at certain times, our behaviour patterns and social interactions will indicate the ego state that is predominant at that time. To take this further, when a patient attends for dental treatment or you are about to carry out that treatment, the words you use, your body language and your behaviour can be identified as being an increment of your current ego state.

Berne also recognised that in a social interaction the *transactions* occur in chains. As he put it, a transactional stimulus from X elicits a transactional response from Y, which in turn becomes a stimulus for X, and so on.

So in the example of the patient–dentist relationship both will begin the interaction in a certain predominant ego state, and these may or may not match with one another. The dynamics of the relationship will influence the direction that the interaction takes, and the predominant ego states of both participants will feed back into these dynamics as further stimuli as the relationship develops.

According to the model, successful communication results from compatible roles of the participants, so the aim in taking a patient-centred approach would be towards both the health professional and the patient adopting the adult role. However, in the paternalistic model described above the professional would be acting in the parent role and in that instance successful communication would result only if the patient were prepared to accept the child role. This may be appropriate in certain circumstances. In a case where the patient is very distressed, for example, this may be the model that comes into play.

Four models of the dentist-patient relationship

As part of the analysis of the process of communication certain styles have been identified which may correspond to the type of relationship occurring between the participants[10].

1) Paternalistic

This relationship in many ways resembles that of a parent and a child, and provided both participants fall easily into their roles this model can be managed successfully, enabling treatment to be carried out comfortably for both parties.

In the relationship the patient tends to play a passive role and the dentist, as an expert, will gain his information from the patient by means of quite specific closed questions. The dentist will then examine the dental area before deciding on the appropriate treatment, which the patient will follow unquestioningly.

A potential drawback is that the "child" patient may rapidly all too easily develop a dependency upon their "parent" dentist, and even tend to regress further into their child mode by becoming readily tearful and difficult to treat.

Historically this relationship was by far the most common in dealings between lay people and professionals including, for example, dentists, doctors and lawyers. Now, with the blurring of professional boundaries, and in an age of fast-developing consumerism and easy availability of information from the Internet and from books and magazines, many patients are becoming "experts", and there may be areas of disagreement or conflict emanating from disparate knowledge and beliefs.

> John was a very successful and aggressive businessman who through his imposing size tended to dominate the room when he came for his regular dental treatment. One morning as I arrived for work I saw his expensive company car parked outside the practice, and as I entered I could hear his angry voice complaining loudly. It turned out that he had chipped an anterior tooth, making it somewhat unsightly. He had a board meeting that morning and was concerned about his appearance, and wanted his dental problem dealt with immediately. My nurse and receptionist were obviously intimidated by him, and I could easily have reacted in the same way. Instead, almost subconsciously, I perceived him as an angry child and went into parent mode, even though I had to look up to him as he towered above me! I heard my voice say quietly, in a caring way, *"Oh dear John, what a shame to have done that. It must be so hard to deal with it. Never mind, we'll be able to sort it out for you and it'll be as good as new, and for now I can smooth it off so it'll look just fine for your meeting."*
>
> To my relief John immediately fell into "child" mode and became almost tearful in his thanks and his apologies to my staff, and even brought them a box of chocolates when he turned up for his appointment for the permanent restoration of the tooth. From then on, our relationship regained its previous adult–adult basis.

2) Mutual

In this model patient and dentist share what is in effect an "adult to adult" relationship. In other words there is a cultural shift away from the paradigm of the passive role of the patient and the authority of the dentist. Increasingly the principal's first name is used as the natural form of address, and a secretary may answer a request for an appointment by saying, "Mary will be able to see you at 3.30 p.m. tomorrow."

In parallel with this aspect of social evolution is the fact that patients have increasing access to information through the press and the Internet, and take a much more active role in their own health care. Further, financial implications increasingly play a much larger part within treatment planning than they may have done historically, and patients will often display interests and have a strong input into discussions involving any projected dental treatment.

Within a mutual relationship the dentist will recognise the importance the patient's beliefs and knowledge play in determining the relationship and the treatment.

Joan, a regular dental patient, was somewhat overweight and was going through a period of depression. She had been told by a lay "specialist" that her problems were caused by a number of allergies, and that she should she have all her many amalgam fillings replaced by composite resin, even dictating in a written note the order in which I should do this. I told Joan in simple terms that my clinical judgement was that her restorations were in good order and that some of the larger amalgams were subgingival, not lending themselves to replacement by composite. I also explained tactfully why I believed the specialist's rationale to be flawed, adding my view that the amount of mercury vapour likely to be released in replacing the fillings would be significant and should be taken into account.

We agreed to a compromise by which I would restore in composite any fillings that *I* felt could be replaced clinically satisfactorily. When I saw Joan a few weeks later, after having replaced only two restorations, she was glowing with health and self-confidence, had lost weight and said that she felt absolutely wonderful. I did not suggest that this might have been a placebo response, but merely congratulated her on her dramatic improvement. No further restorations were needed.

---

3) Consumerist

In a consumer-orientated society, financial factors must inevitably play a role in treatment planning. In addition the influences of a "patient charter" and individual rights, together with increased emphasis upon patient choice, have brought about a change in the relationship between dentist and patient.

Major aspects of this are evident in the fact that many patients will now "shop around", and there is an expectation by the patient of a high level of investigation and information provision, of risk assessment and of acceptable quality of treatment, with litigation becoming an increasingly possible outcome in the case of failure.

Mr Jones was an overbearing, highly successful and well-known local solicitor, approaching retirement. He attended the mixed NHS/private practice, telling the new young associate that he wanted a new full set of dentures made privately, and he wanted the very best. The associate was nervous about mentioning the likely cost but went ahead with the treatment, ultimately fitting the dentures, which met with Mr Jones's delight in every way. Mr Jones then asked for his bill. Only at this stage did the associate nervously suggest an amount, and this fell well *below* the price that Mr Jones had expected to pay.

Mr Jones's attitude changed dramatically, and he said, *"Didn't I tell you I wanted the best? I might just as well have had them done on the NHS!"* He then complained about the fit, the occlusion and the appearance, said that the dentures were unsatisfactory, and stormed out without paying.

The associate was devastated but had learned many useful lessons from the experience.

4) "Default"

In the default model, communication of both information and feelings is poor, leading to a frustrating and unsuccessful interaction. Characteristically, the dentist cannot find the reason for the patient's symptom and the patient, expecting an answer, is confused. The normal sequence can then be a series of referrals and investigations where no individual takes responsibility for addressing any underlying issue.

Enid, a regular patient at the practice, attended as an emergency with severe toothache in the upper left quadrant. In the waiting room she told the receptionist, whom she knew socially, about her many current problems at home.

On examination no teeth were sensitive to hot, cold or percussion, and no pathology was apparent on X-ray. However, on Enid's desperate plea a filling was removed from a tooth and a sedative dressing inserted. Over the next three months this pattern was repeated, and eventually several teeth were root-filled, but still the problem persisted. Ultimately the dentist–patient relationship became severely frayed and tense and Enid was referred to the local dental hospital where there was a similar lack of success in identifying the cause of her pain.

At about the same time the situation at Enid's home became untenable and her medical GP diagnosed depression. Enid entered counselling and was prescribed antidepressants. The toothache vanished overnight. Enid expressed her dissatisfaction with her dental treatment to all and sundry and, to mutual relief, moved to another dental practice.

Having established rapport with the patient, moving on to the use of hypnosis to facilitate treatment becomes a natural development of the professional relationship.

4

Demystifying Hypnosis

Trust

Trust is an essential element underlying the successful use of hypnosis in practice. The patient has to trust the dentist. It could be argued that this trust is implicit in that the patient is prepared to submit to having dental treatment by that same dentist. However, a patient about to consent to hypnosis may feel they are taking a great leap into the unknown, and may have many anxieties about taking this leap. If the patient has, for example, seen a performance of stage hypnosis in which the volunteers on stage, apparently under the influence and control of the hypnotist, made fools of themselves, they may equate hypnosis with a loss of control.

An anxious or fearful patient may be unable to trust not only the dentist, but also themselves. They may doubt that they have the ability or psychological makeup to use hypnosis successfully, or their self-esteem may be so low that any success can seem quite beyond them.

Popular culture

Because the word "hypnosis" is used in many different contexts, encompassing not only entertainment but also literature and films, the majority of ideas and concepts about hypnosis held by the public may be flawed and inaccurate. The concept that hypnosis can be a valuable adjunct to medical and dental treatment might initially seem strange to the patient.

Two of the main misconceptions fostered by popular culture are that hypnosis involves the loss of control over one's actions and that it has amazing and supernatural powers. Not infrequently the word will bring to mind images of Rasputin, the sinister, shadowy figure behind the throne of pre-Revolution Russia[11], or of Svengali, the evil anti-hero of George Du Maurier's nineteenth-century novel *Trilby*[12]. The myth is perpetuated in the TV science fiction series *The X Files*[13], where hypnosis is used to recover memories of alien abduction.

Counteracting misconceptions

Because of the references in literature to power and control issues surrounding hypnosis, it is obviously important that the dentist using hypnosis is able to correct any misconceptions the patient may have. Giving an accurate description of how easy and pleasant the process of entering hypnosis will be, together with the likely benefits of treatment, is essential before treatment starts.

In fact the concept that hypnosis involves domination by the hypnotist is far from the truth. One aim of the use of hypnosis in dental treatment is to increase the patient's own control over their thoughts, feelings and behaviour. In addition research has confirmed that people will not do anything in hypnosis that they would not do while awake and, if pressed, will come out of hypnosis and refuse to cooperate[14].

Although positive expectations are usually necessary for people to experience hypnosis[15], the belief that hypnosis will provide miraculous cures for all their problems is not helpful. It is important that the patient understands that they must play an active part in the process, with the hypnotist acting as a guide and teacher. The success of hypnotic treatment depends on the patient responding to suggestions and then acting upon them. A useful model to explain this would be that of taking tennis or piano lessons. The coach or tutor can suggest various ways to make real and sustained improvements, but it is the learner's responsibility to incorporate those skills and abilities into their performance. Similarly when these skills and abilities have become "programmed" into that person's performance they become natural and are used quite unconsciously.

Historically the word "hypnosis" has been associated with sleep or even unconsciousness and there will be patients who believe this still to be the case, so it is essential that the patient understands that they will remain aware of what is happening and will remember any suggestions. You can reassure them that were they to be asleep they would not be able to respond, and as a result would not benefit from the therapeutic session. You might also tell the patient that hypnosis is not an "all or nothing" state and that it can vary from person to person, and even in an individual from day to day, but that everyone can gain a benefit from it, and with practice it becomes easier.

It might be helpful to compare hypnosis to experiences that people have in their day-to-day lives, like daydreaming or becoming so absorbed in a book or film that everything else fades into the background. These realistic expectations can forestall the patient from thinking that the hypnosis did not work because they expected something more remarkable to happen. Using the word "trance" has also been shown sometimes to impair the patient's response to suggestions, possibly again because their initial expectations have been flawed[16].

You might describe hypnosis as a state of mind that allows appropriate suggestions to be acted on much more powerfully than usual. It is as though helpful suggestions are registered without the usual conscious censorship, criticism or self-doubt.

A script for explaining hypnosis to patients in order to give them a positive mind-set may be something like this:

"You've probably been in a daydreamy state very similar to hypnosis many times every day of your life. Can you recall how sometimes as you wake up in the morning it's as though you remain half asleep, and thoughts and fantasies just seem to drift through your head, until you say to yourself 'I've got to get up!', and reality breaks back into your mind.

Or I wonder whether you have ever been so absorbed in a film or a book that the outside world seemed to fade away ... you knew it was there, and if an emergency had cropped up you would have responded to it ... but it was easier just to let your mind and your imagination become really deeply involved and your awareness of the outside world grow less and less ... and you got so involved in the film or book that it seemed to become almost real ...

Or maybe you've been driving the car on a familiar journey and been so involved in your thoughts, or listening to the radio or music, that you were barely conscious that you were driving the car ... people sometimes say 'it was as if the car had driven itself', or 'my mind was miles away'... so that when you arrived at your destination you could not remember anything of the journey. And yet at the same time you had been driving safely, changing gear and stopping at red lights, without any conscious memory of having done so.

Hypnosis is a safe natural process, very similar to daydreaming or being absorbed in a book or film. During hypnosis you will probably feel very physically relaxed and comfortable, and most people describe being in hypnosis as a very pleasant experience.

Hypnosis is a way of allowing yourself to act on appropriate suggestions without the usual self doubt and worry getting in the way. You can find that your attention is much more focused so that the therapy or treatment can be more effective.

So you won't be asleep or unconscious, and you will be in control at all times. Should you wish to, you will be able to speak or cough or move around in the chair normally without disturbing the hypnosis, and you may come out of hypnosis whenever you wish to do so. You'll probably be aware of what's going on around you, but happier simply to ignore it.

People respond to hypnosis in different ways. You may feel heavy and reluctant to move, or possibly light and floaty. What is important is that hypnosis can be a very powerful way for you to gain control over your thoughts, feelings or emotions.

I am here to help you get the maximum benefit from your hypnosis sessions, so please feel free to ask any questions before we start."

Much time can be saved by designing user-friendly patient information leaflets, and an example is given in the Appendix.

Finally, avoid challenge situations with patients; if a person says "I bet you can't hypnotise me!" they will almost certainly be right! The patient's motivation and trust is of paramount importance. If they are motivated *not* to enter hypnosis, that is precisely what they will achieve.

5

Stage Hypnosis

The view of hypnosis shared by a number of prospective patients will have been formed by having seen a TV or stage show, and many people find it difficult to reconcile the serious and valuable use of hypnosis in a clinical setting such as dentistry with their perception of its frivolous nature and the strange antics of the "performers" in the stage show.

The law

The Hypnotism Act (1952) was an attempt to regulate the use of hypnosis when used for entertainment. In summary, the Act gives local authorities the power to grant to places already licensed for public entertainment power to attach "conditions regulating or prohibiting the giving of an exhibition, demonstration or performance of hypnotism on any person at the place to which the licence is granted".

The Act prohibits any "exhibition, demonstration or performance of hypnotism as entertainment to which the public are admitted ... whether on payment or otherwise, without such authorisation", but makes an exception when the hypnotism takes place during the course of a play.

It also prohibits the use of hypnotism as entertainment on any person below the age of eighteen.

The concerns

If hypnosis is seen as a way of coercing people into carrying out bizarre acts and making fools of themselves many who could genuinely benefit from its use in medical and dental situations will be deterred.

Some of the audience may be suffering from psychiatric disorders - a contraindication to hypnosis unless carried out by a specialist practitioner. (see Appendix). In addi-

tion, anyone who is feeling ill, or fearful and anxious can have times of emotional fragili-
ty and vulnerability. In hypnosis such emotions can come to the surface quite readily.
In the safety of the consulting room and a warm, trusting relationship with the therapist this can often be helpful, and a responsible therapist will always allow the patient
time to return gently to "here and now" feeling calm and secure again. Because in stage
hypnosis there is no monitoring of the participants' state of mind, a volunteer who has
a psychiatric illness or is going through a fragile emotional spell is extremely vulnera-
ble. Susceptible members of the audience may also be drawn into the hypnotic experience, and again there is no monitoring of their response and its potential after-effects.
Furthermore, in stage hypnosis there is no follow-up afterwards to check participants'
emotional state, a routine procedure within clinical hypnosis.

In clinical hypnosis the alerting procedure is integral to the whole experience, and will
always be conducted with extreme care and caution (see Chapter 9). In contrast, "wak-
ening" the patient on stage is often very abruptly carried out. For example, it is docu-
mented that a performer in a public house show terminated the trance experience for
his volunteers by suggesting that when he said "goodnight" the subjects would feel 10,000
volts of electricity through the seat of their chairs[17]. At the very least such an alerting
process may lead to profound confusion and disorientation of the participants.

Other concerns relate to alteration of sensation and to post-hypnotic suggestions. In clinical practice it is fundamental that such suggestions are removed or are time and situation
limited, and that the patient's response to this is checked out thoroughly afterwards.
Alteration in sensation is a key ingredient of stage hypnosis, and all too often reversal of
any change does not take place, and participants may again be left feeling very confused.

In a similar vein, the use of post-hypnotic suggestions is central to hypnosis when used
in a clinical situation. For example, in dental practice a common post-hypnotic suggestion
may be that the next time the patient comes for treatment they will go into deep relaxation
as soon as they sit in the dental chair. Note that this suggestion is situation and time limited. In stage hypnosis the post-hypnotic suggestion may be that when the band plays a certain tune the subject will fall asleep, and there often will be no attempt made to reverse the
suggestion, yet again possibly leading to a confused and disorientated subject.

What happens in a stage hypnosis performance?

While there are divided opinions as to how much of the behaviour of the volunteers on
stage is due to hypnosis and how much to role play, what is undoubtedly true is that
many of the skills inherent in stage hypnosis presentation are in showmanship, in the
selection of suitable volunteers, and in rapid induction techniques.

Selection of volunteers
Following a series of simple psychological tricks aimed at establishing rapport with the
audience and at the same time demonstrating his own credentials as a hypnotist, the per-

former will introduce a "hypnotisability test" by which his potential volunteers will be identified. This test may be to ask his audience to clasp their hands tightly together over their heads, and try as hard as possible to separate their hands. While they are struggling the performer will build on the belief and expectation of the audience, exhorting them that those of the audience who are not able to separate their hands however hard they try are excellent hypnotic subjects. By this time many of the audience will have realised that the reason their hands won't separate is simply that their knuckles are locked together, and so by relaxing slightly find that they can drop their hands down again.

Invitation onto the stage

The stage hypnotist will then invite any of the "good hypnotic subjects" who wish to take part in the show to come up onto the stage. The dozen or so people who mount the stage will each be invited by the hypnotist to stand in front in one of the chairs ranged along the back of the stage, and the hypnotist will quietly ascertain that they are happy to take part in the show. On their acquiescence typically he will place his hand on their forehead, say "Just drop your hands and go to sleep", and gently push them back into the chair where, characteristically they will one by one appear to go to sleep.

Suggestion

At this stage the hypnotist will probably have his back to the audience as he concentrates upon the volunteers, but he will also be playing to the audience over his shoulder, indirectly bringing the pressure of the audience to bear on the suggestions that he now makes to each of the volunteers. The suggestions will range extremely widely in bizarre inventiveness and detail but will be appropriate to each volunteer's degree of exhibitionism, and will generally involve a number of post-hypnotic suggestions aimed at entertaining the audience.

Stage hypnosis and clinical hypnosis

Of the many ingredients that go into the successful relationship between hypnotist and subject, or in the case of dentistry between dentist and patient, certain key elements should be present. On the part of the subject/patient, Gindes[18] identified *belief, expectation* and *misdirection of attention*, together with the individual's *imagination*[18]. To these we must add *motivation* as a prime and overriding influence.

Audience and prospective volunteers see the adverts and buy tickets and believe and expect the excitement of a night out, seeing at one and the same time a form of entertainment that is mystical, bizarre, funny and apparently uninhibited. A number of the people going to the show will be out for a good time with friends, and challenges such as "I bet you daren't go up on stage!" will abound. Among the audience, too, there will be a mixture of belief systems relating to hypnosis; there will be those with a genuine interest and a sprinkling of sceptics.

The skill of the stage hypnotist is in the ability to gain rapid and powerful rapport with his audience and potential volunteers; building upon their positive beliefs and expectations; ensuring the self-selection of volunteer performers, who thus demonstrate their motivation to come on stage; having the "gift of the gab" in setting up imaginary tasks for the volunteers and art of showmanship in using the audience responses to build upon a volunteer's imaginary situation.

If we look at Gindes's model in terms of the anxious and fearful dental patient, we can perceive a very different state of affairs. Beliefs and expectations may include insights of their own powerlessness in the feared relationship with a powerful dentist; an expectation of bad news, of loss of control, of pain and discomfort and of making a fool of themselves. Their imagination may be running amok following earlier experiences, others' stories and the folklore of dentistry, and the smells, sounds, sights and sensations experienced at your practice. They may also be ignorant of what is to happen and therefore highly anxious about the use of hypnosis.

In your favour is the fact that, for whatever reason, the patient must have been sufficiently motivated to make their appointment and actually turn up, so this may be a factor on which you base your very necessary rapid rapport-building. From the stage hypnotist you can learn the vital importance of presentation, an environment conducive to rapport-building, good interpersonal relationships and positive use of the patient's imagination and motivation.

Summary

While there is considerable debate upon the actual physical and psychological harm that stage hypnosis may cause to volunteers, what is without doubt is that among clinicians there is almost universal condemnation of hypnosis as a stage act. This is primarily because the distorted image of hypnosis portrayed on the stage may well leave potential patients with a false impression and build upon their fears that hypnosis is a state in which they will be controlled by the hypnotist and made to carry out silly and possibly dangerous acts. Thus people who could gain hugely from hypnosis within dentistry may be deterred and thus forfeit that benefit.

6

Communicating with Patients

Whether or not you propose to introduce hypnosis into a patient's treatment, a detailed and carefully taken history will greatly improve the prospect of a successful intervention. Information gathered will give you insights into the patient's concerns, helping you to formulate an effective treatment plan.

In addition, details may well emerge that suggest the imagery and metaphors you might wish to introduce within hypnosis. Importantly, the way in which you elicit their history from a patient will have a large influence on the rapport that develops between you.

The initial part of your history-taking will inevitably be concentrating upon the presenting dental concerns of the patient. When using hypnosis as part of the management of those concerns, certain key factors should also be determined.

Active listening

In their song "The Sound of Silence"[19] Simon and Garfunkle describe "people hearing without listening", and all of us are guilty of this from time to time, particularly when a patient is giving us their history and we are busy working out when it will be appropriate to interrupt, and what we are going to say next.

A patient revealing their history is giving much more than a simple narrative. It is important that you are aware of the sense of what is being imparted and the actual words the patient uses, but in addition a vast amount of information is being given by the manner in which the words are expressed and by the way that this relates to the patient's body language.

Is there congruence between what the patient says and the way that he says it? Does the person appear quite proud to claim "I bet I'm the worst patient you've ever had", or "I bet you've never seen a mouth as bad as mine"? When a patient says "I'm really scared", what exactly is it that they are scared of?

Obtaining accurate information

Before thinking about how you yourself communicate, it is important to consider what the patient is communicating to *you*. This is your opportunity to get to know the patient, their wants, needs and feelings, rather than seeing them simply as a collection of medical conditions and dental diseases.

The initial part of your history taking will inevitably be concentrating upon the presenting dental concerns of the patient. When you are planning to use hypnosis certain key factors should also be determined.

Within the history-taking, ask the patient whether they have had hypnosis before in any context. If, for example, they have used hypnosis successfully in smoking cessation, you may use this experience as a model for the style of hypnosis that you will use.

An enquiry into past dental experiences, especially in early childhood, may have relevance to present perceptions and behaviour, and an outline of the patient's work and hobbies may open up avenues for the later use of imagery.

It is also helpful to investigate any stressful situations and events that the patient has encountered, and any way in which this is currently affecting them.

Any patient who is taking consciousness-altering drugs or who has a psychiatric illness should be referred to a suitably experienced therapist with specialist training, as any effects of hypnosis will be unpredictable (see Appendix).

You need to obtain *accurate* information from patients in order to treat them effectively, safely and appropriately. It is worth remembering here that the anxiety and fear response impairs cognitive functioning. This may frequently be seen in a nervous patient's inability to express themselves concisely in presentation of their concerns, and likewise an inability for them to understand and to take on board your explanations and description of the clinical situation and any proposed treatment plan.

We all appreciate being listened to when we divulge our concerns and worries, and so the patient needs to *know* that they have been listened to and that their story has been heard and affirmed. *Active listening* is a way to ensure that this happens.

Sit in the optimum position as described earlier and establish eye contact, at the same time allowing both the patient and yourself the option of breaking this eye contact. Open the exchange with a greeting and always use the patient's preferred name. Find out what the patient thinks they are making the visit for, and note that this is not necessarily what *you* think they are there for!

Affirmation

As the patient gives their story, concentrate upon what they are saying, the way in which they are saying it, their corresponding facial expression and their body language.

Constantly affirm and validate their statements by appropriate responses such as, reflection of expression, (restrained) nods of agreement, para-verbal responses such as *"mmm…, ah-ah…"*, verbal responses such as *"yes, I know what you mean"*, and occasionally reflecting back by validating or repeating the patient's words. Again, note the patient's response to affirmation. If the ploy is overused, the effect can easily become irritating and appear false.

Reflection

Reflection can be an effective way of encouraging the patient to expand their story, at the same time indicating active listening and increasing rapport.

For example, if the patient is obviously upset and says, "I can't believe that I need some teeth out", you might respond by:

- reflecting back the patient's own words: "You can't believe it."
- an interpretation of the words: "I guess it's too much to take in."
- acknowledgement of the patient's feeling: "You feel shocked."

As it is important that the patient can perceive that you are involved in listening, notes should not be taken at this time, but can be made later.

Silence

Silence is a valuable tool that is much underused. The patient may take considerable time to process a statement or question you have put to them, possibly because they are disturbed by it or possibly because they are upset and struggling to find and articulate the right response. It is important that you allow them time to respond without barging in with a further question.

Sometimes a reflective remark such as "you seem pretty upset" will validate them and help them to clarify their thoughts.

Paralinguistic features

The way in which you deliver your words will have a profound impact upon their meaning to the recipient. Modification in volume, tone, pitch, inflection and speed of delivery can have an effect as powerful as the actual words you use. For example, the phrase "you brushed your teeth today" might be construed as a statement of fact, a sarcastic remark, an expression of surprise and congratulation or a question, depending upon inflection and tone.

Open and closed questions

At times you will need to question the patient in order to clarify points and to guide them into giving necessary and specific information. The style of the questioning you employ may be *open* or *closed*.

An open question is one that allows discretion and freedom in the way it is answered and might be used to elicit the patient's feelings, emotions and beliefs, letting you obtain the full story as the patient sees it.

Examples are "how are you feeling today?" or "what seems to be the trouble?" or "how do you feel about having crowns on your front teeth?"

The patient is thus invited to give a narrative answer through which a number of important clues to their problems and concerns might emerge.

A closed question, on the other hand, is designed to elicit a one- or two-word answer and is valuable when you are attempting to clarify detail.

Generally closed questions fall into three types:

- an item of detail: "When did the pain start?"
- a choice of alternatives: "Is it dull or sharp?"
- a yes/no response: "Does it still hurt?"

Both forms of questioning can be valuable, but in the early stages of a conversation open questions will provide the most information and give a greater insight into the patient's condition and situation. Closed questions should be reserved as requests for very specific information, such as "Have you ever been diagnosed with a heart murmur?"

The closed question is used frequently in hypnosis, particularly with reference to the ideomotor response (see Chapter 14), as generally the patient is so comfortable and relaxed that they have little inclination to expand on a response to a question, and the effort involved would probably disturb the hypnosis.

The language we use

Language is not merely a medium for transferring ideas from one mind to another. Our meaning is complicated by context, tone of voice, previous experience and power relations, among other factors. Hypnosis is grounded in the use of language and suggestions, so training in its use can make us conscious of the words that we use in everyday communication. Every word or sentence that we use can be understood as a suggestion and if we are aware of the possible effects we can change the nature of the communication. Equally, by being unaware of the use and power of language we can destroy with one word all the rapport we have painstakingly built up with a patient.

Forewarning the patient

Dentists and staff will often prepare patients for potential procedural discomfort with descriptions of the possible pain or undesirable experience, feeling that this practice is compassionate and helpful. The authors share the belief that the effect of using such language may, on the contrary, serve to increase anxiety and apprehension, and a recent study[20] supports this view.

In a three-arm prospective randomised trial, the interactions of 159 patients with their health-care providers during interventional radiological procedures were video-taped and analysed. For the Standard Group of patients, specialist nurses were instructed to behave normally, do their best to comfort the patient, but abstain from induction of imagery and hypnosis. In the Attention Group verbal and non-verbal behaviour were prescribed, and encompassed such behaviours as matching the patient's non-verbal communication pattern, attentive listening, provision of perception of control and avoidance of negatively loaded suggestions.

The study showed that warning the patient of pain or undesirable experiences resulted in increased pain and anxiety, and sympathising with the patient in such terms after a painful event did not increase reported pain but resulted in greater anxiety.

The conclusion was that, contrary to common belief, warning or sympathising by using language that refers to negative experiences may not make patients feel better.

Always use positive language

Consider what happens when you read the phrase "don't think of a pink elephant". Inevitably your mind ignores the word "don't" and processes the object of the sentence. In order not to think of a pink elephant you first construct the image, and then find yourself working out ways of making it disappear.

You may be asking yourself the relevance of pink elephants to a book on hypnosis in dentistry, and the reply is that this simple strategy of eliminating negatives can be a tool by which you reconstruct your entire mode of communication with patients at your practice. Negative language is not simply words such as "no" and "nothing". A negative word is any word that communicates to the recipient a negative affect or emotion. And such negative words as "pain", "fear", "hurt", "forceps" and "surgery" can too easily colour your working vocabulary.

Heightened suggestibility is intrinsic both to deep relaxation and to the state of anxiety and tension. As that anxious patient sits in your reception room or your surgery he is subjected to a vast range of stimuli, which he perceives as negative and which, because of his heightened state of suggestibility superimposed on his previous experiences and perceptual processing, may serve only to increase his fear and anxiety.

Explain what the patient may feel, and not what they will *not* feel. For example, within the dental situation the often-used phrase "this won't hurt" takes on a new and unintended meaning. This could be rephrased effectively to *"as you relax, this will feel much more comfortable for you".*

In particular, avoid the phrase "you won't feel anything". This is untrue, as the patient inevitably will feel *something*; the only times one feels nothing at all is when one is unconscious or dead. If you tell a patient that they won't feel anything, then the sensations of dental treatment are likely to be perceived as unpleasant or as pain, rather than as the vibration or the coolness by which you might characterise them.

Framing

This well-known phenomenon affects the decisions people make based on the way that options are presented to them. It has been investigated in several choices about a range of issues and with people from all walks of life[21].

Maybe you can associate this concept with the way you might present a treatment plan to a patient. Study the two following examples and decide which way you would choose to present this situation to a dental patient.

You have broken a tooth and your dentist tells you about a new treatment that aims to save broken teeth. He says that the treatment has a 60% chance of saving the tooth. In other words, six out of ten broken teeth treated will last for about five years. The treatment costs twice as much as having the tooth taken out.

What would you choose to do?
Alternative A: Have the treatment carried out.
Alternative B: Have the tooth taken out.

You have broken a tooth and your dentist tells you about a new treatment that aims to save broken teeth. He says that the treatment has a 40% chance of failure. In other words, four out of ten broken teeth treated will have to be extracted. The remainder last for about five years. The treatment costs twice as much as having the tooth taken out.

What would you choose to do?
Alternative A: Have the treatment carried out.
Alternative B: Have the tooth taken out.

Obviously, we cannot escape this effect, but once aware of it we can use it positively for the benefit of our patients. The power of framing and reframing messages in a positive way must not be underestimated.

Dental language

Think back to when you were a student. Before you actually filled any teeth you learned an entirely new language with unfamiliar words: mesial, distal, occlusal. You learned to say cavity instead of hole and restoration rather than filling. You learned dental jargon.

Unfortunately, too many dentists expect their patients to understand this language without the benefit of a similar university education. This can lead to misunderstandings and patients feeling that you are "talking over their heads" and being secretive. Of course, if the patient is an adult you must avoid the related mistake of being patronising and talking down to them.

At the same time there is within our language an element of familiarity, breeding a certain casual acceptance. We are used to words such as "extraction" and "injection", and can easily ignore the impact that these words will have upon an anxious patient. This whole situation is compounded by a fact referred to earlier in this section, in that because of their physiological arousal the anxious patient will not be in a position to comprehend a complex treatment plan, and will be in a state of hyper-suggestibility, further potentiating the damage caused by ill-chosen words.

Within the practice it is wise to train your entire staff in the use of simple euphemisms so that words such as "forceps" and "drill" and "hypodermic" become redundant. Thus you will find that the use of hypnosis in dentistry will impact positively your behaviour, your use of words and the entire ambience of your working situation.

Touch

Because of the nature of dentistry, you spend almost all your professional life touching your patients, and yet the quandary of appropriate and inappropriate touch needs to be a constant consideration.

Touch can be *facilitative*. For example, we may shake a person's hand in greeting or in parting as a way of establishing a relationship. We obviously use *functional* touch when we are palpating a gland or actually filling teeth, whereas *therapeutic* touch can happen almost intuitively when we touch a distressed patient on the shoulder or arm as a way of communicating understanding, support and reassurance. However, fine judgement must be used here as a number of patients may find such touch to be inappropriate, and indeed we should constantly monitor the patient's non-verbal cues in order to prevent misunderstandings occurring.

Any touch that creates uncertainty in the patient's mind will inevitably act as a block against successful rapport and hypnosis. Inevitably such uncertainty will be increased when you are working with a patient whose eyes are closed.

In this context, as in many others, the importance of the presence of a chaperone can not be over-emphasised.

Summarising

Summarising draws together the *significant* aspects of the interaction. You may summarise your understanding of the patient's symptoms, feeling and point of view, and the key points of the treatment proposed. This gives an opportunity for both you and the patient to clarify any misrepresentations and misunderstandings.

Your summarising should be clearly stated, but a slightly questioning tone in your voice will encourage the patient to clarify their view.

Explaining

The ability to deliver a lucid, coherent explanation is critical in enabling the patient to understand their problem, diagnosis and potential treatment plan. An explanation should be clear and easily understandable, bearing in mind the patient's intellect, level of knowledge of the subject, emotional state and needs at that time.

The explanation should:

- use a series of logical points
- avoid or explain any jargon
- repeat and emphasise key points
- use examples and diagrams
- give specific rather than vague advice
- check out the patient's understanding by asking for feedback.

So now you have created the situation of comfort, rapport and trust between yourself, your practice and the patient. It is a natural continuum to move from here into hypnosis, and this is what we will be doing in the next chapters.

References

1. Atterbury R. The use of verbal relaxation therapy for sedation during dental therapy. Anaesthesia Progress 1984;31(1):27–30.
2. Taylor S. Music in general hospital treatment 1900–1950. J Music Ther 1981;18(2):62–73.
3. At Charing Cross Hospital in London. New Sci 1983;1339(20).
4. Standley J. Music as a therapeutic intervention in medical and dental treatment: research and clinical applications. In: Wigram T, Saperson B, West R, eds. The Art and Science of Music Therapy: A Handbook. Switzerland: Harwood Academic Publications, 1995.
5. Campbell D. The Mozart Effect. London: Hodder & Stoughton, 1997.
6. Gottlieb B. Sound Therapy. New Choices in Natural Healing, p. 127. Emmaus, PA: Rodale Press, 1995.
7. Chu S, Downes JJ. Odour-evoked autobiographical memories: psychological investigations of the Proustian phenomena. Chem Senses 2000;25:111–16.
8. Robin O, Alaoui-Ismaili O, Dittman A, Vernett-Maury E. Emotional responses evoked by dental odors: an evaluation from autonomic parameters. J Dent Res 1998;77(8):1638–46.
9. Berne E. Transactional Analysis in Psychotherapy. New York: Grove Press, 1961.
10. Alder B, Porter M, Abraham C, van Teijlingen, E. Psychology and Sociology Applied to Medicine. 2nd Ed. Edinburgh: Churchill Livingstone, 2004.
11. DeJonge A. Life and Times of Grigori Rasputin. New York: Dorset Press, 1987.
12. DuMaurier G. Trilby. Oxford: OUP, 1998.
13. Bowman R. The X Files. UK: BBC TV, 1998.
14. Shor RE, Orne, MT. The Nature of Hypnosis. Berkeley, CA: University of California, 1959.
15. Spanos NP, Burnley MC, Cross PA. Response expectancies and interpretations as determinants of hypnotic responding. J Pers Soc Psychol 1993 Dec. 65(6):1237–42.
16. Kirsch I, Braffman W. Correlates of hypnotizability: The first empirical study. Contemporary Hypnosis 1999;16(4): 224–30.
17. O'Keefe T. Investigating Stage Hypnosis. London: Extraordinary People Press, 1998.
18. Gindes B. New Concepts of Hypnosis: Theories, Techniques and Practical Applications. Chatsworth, CA: Wilshire Book Company, 1951.
19. Simon P. The Sound of Silence. Sounds of Silence, 1966.
20. Lang EV, Hatsiopoulou O, T. Koch, Berbaum K, Lutgendorf S, Kettenmann E, et al. Can words hurt? Patient-provider interactions during invasive procedures. J Pain 2005;Mar. 114(1–2):303–9.
21. Tversky A, D. Kahneman. The framing of decisions and the psychology of choice. Science 1981;211(30).

For further and more detailed study of stage hypnosis and possible adverse effects of hypnosis, it is recommended that you read: Hartland's Medical and Dental Hypnosis. 4th Ed. London: Churchill Livingstone, 2002, pp. 480–8.

7

Induction

Induction is the process by which a patient "enters" hypnosis. The induction process itself is not hypnosis but it represents the starting point of the hypnotic intervention. You will learn in the following chapter of strategies for *deepening* hypnosis. Deepening normally follows induction, the two processes interacting as a continuum, and certain induction techniques are indistinguishable from those used for the deepening process.

It will be assumed in the following section you have established rapport with the patient, have explained the nature of hypnosis, have discussed and resolved any of the patient's doubts and fears regarding hypnosis, and have agreed with them that hypnosis is an appropriate tool in managing the next part of their dental treatment.

You should appear confident, yet not over confident, and should speak quite slowly, quietly and evenly. It is helpful to explain to the patient that they will probably feel that they could open their eyes at any time during hypnosis, but that the state is so comfortable that it will be more pleasant to allow them to stay closed. You can tell them that the state is like a daydream in which they will be aware of everything around them but happier to stay within the daydream. Encourage the patient to let things happen "of their own accord', and not bother to "try" to do anything at all.

There are innumerable methods of induction, both formal and informal, and as you gain experience you will have a number of these at your disposal, tailoring your technique to the needs of the patient.

Most formal induction procedures commence with suggestions of physical tension, commonly around the eyes, eyelids or limbs. The patient is encouraged to direct their attention to the area while suggestions are given for release of that tension.

Introducing induction

A valuable aid to successful induction is firstly to demonstrate to the patient what you as a therapist will be asking him to do.

> *"In a few moments I will be asking you roll your eyes upwards and then to close your eyes. Shortly after that I will be asking you to hold your breath, and then, as you let the breath out, to let yourself become deeply relaxed ... now if you'll just watch me I'll show you what I expect you to do ..."*

Demonstrate this at the same time as you describe what is expected. Note that when you demonstrate, all actions, and particularly the relaxation, should be *very slightly* exaggerated, in effect giving a pre-hypnotic suggestion that the patient will enter a particularly deep level of relaxation.

Eye fixation upon a pen or a dental mirror handle

Ask the patient to focus their eyes on a pen or the dental mirror that you hold about 30 cm (12 inches) away and level with their eyes. Slowly raise the pen to the level of the top of the patient's head and ask the patient to continue gazing at the pen. After a few seconds slowly move the pen downwards, and as the patient's eyes follow this invite him to close his eyes.

> *"... now ... I'd like you to focus really hard on this pen I'm holding in front of you ... and as I raise it, please follow it with your eyes, all the time keeping your gaze really concentrated hard on it ...* [after about 10 seconds very slowly lower the pen to below the patient's chin level] *... and continue to follow it with your eyes ... until you're possibly feeling your eyes are growing tired ... and your eyelids are getting so heavy ... that they will want to close ... and when that happens, just let your eyes close ... and let yourself just let go ... and feel yourself sinking down into the chair as you relax more and more deeply ..."*

Simple eye roll

This is a rapid method that is very much suited to dental practice where time may be at a premium. The technique is not suitable for patients who are wearing contact lenses. Dental patients will usually be wearing protective goggles, but if the patient is wearing spectacles he may be given the option of removing them prior to induction.

Ask the patient to roll their eyes upwards, and while the eyes are rolled upwards to close their eyelids over them, keeping their eyes raised. Then ask them to hold their breath for a moment and as they release the breath to relax their eyes and eyelids, allowing the relaxation to flow down through their body on each subsequent outgoing breath.

As an alternative you might ask the patient to follow the eye closure simply by taking three deep breaths and spreading the relaxation down through the body with each exhalation.

Note that this is not the technique of choice for the elderly or for others who may find the eye roll unpleasant or physically difficult to carry out. An alternative is to ask the patient simply to close his eyelids and then to raise his eyes behind the closed eyelids.

> *"... now I wonder if you would roll your eyes upwards ... just as though you're trying to look out of the top of your head ... and, keeping your eyes rolled up, gently close your eyelids over them ... this may seem a little strange but just take your time and let it happen ... that's great ...*
> [characteristically the eyelids will flicker during this manoeuvre and the whites of the eyes will be clearly visible as the eyes close]
> *... and now please take a gentle breath and hold it ... good ... and as you let that breath out allow your eyelids to relax and let your eyes drop to their normal position behind your closed eyelids ... and just let everything go ... and feel yourself sinking down into the chair as you relax more and more deeply ..."*

or

> *"... and now I'd like you to take three deep breaths ... and each time as you let the breath out ... let the relaxation flow down throughout your whole body each time you breathe out ... one ... and two ... and three ... and just let everything go ... and feel yourself sinking down into the chair as you relax more and more deeply ..."*

Fractionated eye closure (after Dave Elman)

Dave Elman was a stage hypnotist in the USA who in the 1950s began demonstrating his techniques to doctors and dentists, and who became recognised as the foremost teacher of hypnosis in the country. Basing his work on his stage act meant that he was concerned with speed and the concept of what he called "selective thinking"[1].

Explain to the patient that you are going to ask them to close their eyes. Now place your hand a few inches above their normal eye level and about 15 cm (6 inches) away from their face. Move your hand downwards in front of their face saying:

> *"... take a long deep breath and close your eyes ... now let those muscles round your eyes relax to the point where they won't work ... test them and make sure they won't work ... test them hard .... that's right! that's very good!"* [you will often see the patient struggling to open their eyes unsuccessfully, at which stage you might simply say the following]
>
> *"... and now you don't even need to test them or try to open them ... just let all that tension go ... and let yourself totally relax ... Now just let that feeling of relaxation go right down to*

> *your toes .... that's fine. Now we'll do that exercise all over again but the next time I ask you to open and close your eyes that lovely feeling of relaxation will be twice as deep as it is now .... twice as deep .... you just let it be like that. Now open your eyes and really let yourself relax, ... close your eyes again .... that's it, very good indeed! and the next time you do this you'll relax even more ... open your eyes .... now close your eyes and experience the wave of relaxation that surges over you ... now I'm going to lift your hand up and let it drop back into your lap .... I want it to be as limp as a dish-rag ... as limp as a rag doll. If you've followed your instructions properly, that relaxation will have gone right down to your toes ... And when I lift your hand up and let it go, it will flop down onto your lap, just let it flop down ... That's right ... now you feel very, very relaxed, physically more relaxed than you've ever been ..."*

Eye fixation and direct suggestion

For this technique you will ask the patient to focus his gaze on a chosen point on the ceiling or wall and then give suggestions geared towards physical relaxation culminating in eye closure.

> *"... please choose a point on the wall or ceiling in front of you ... and slightly above your normal line of vision ... and I'd like you just to gaze at the point and not take your eyes away from it ... and let your hands flop in your lap ... and be aware how comfortable you feel in the chair ... how well supported your neck and shoulders are ... how comfortable your back feels as you let your body just relax into the chair ... but please keep your eyes firmly fixed on that spot ... as you relax ... right down to your ankles ... feet ... toes ... aware of my voice ... aware that your heart beat is becoming comfortable, calm, rhythmic, slow ... your breathing is slower, deeper, calmer, regular ... and as you continue to gaze at that point you are probably aware that your eyes are becoming watery ... it's harder to concentrate on that point ... your eyelids are beginning to flicker ... they feel heavy ... your eyes probably want to close ... maybe it's getting hard to keep them open ... when you're ready to close them you can let them close ... and just let everything go ... and feel yourself sinking down into the chair as you relax more and more deeply ..."*

A "safe place"

This method contains both induction and deepening suggestions, and can be particularly useful for the anxious patient who is apprehensive about suggestions that they feel are too directive. Towards the end of this script you will notice the use of a *post-hypnotic suggestion* (see Chapter 15).

"Now ... what I'd like you to do is simply close your eyes ... and be prepared just to let go ... to let yourself drift along with some ideas and suggestions I'm going to be giving you ...

I wonder if there's a special place where you really love to be ... your own special place ... it might be a real place you've been to ... might be a place you've just heard about and would love to go to ... might be pure fantasy ... it really doesn't matter ... but you know that when you are there you can feel so calm ... so secure ... so relaxed ...
... you might be on your own ... or other people ... special people might be with you ... it doesn't matter ... some people like to relax by being energetic ... by doing all sorts of things ... and others like to be really still and rested ... really peaceful ... it doesn't matter ... and you can just let yourself be there in your mind ... or maybe just watch yourself being there ... like a film or a video in your mind ... it doesn't matter ... and it's just so calm, secure and relaxed ... maybe you can even hear some of the sounds of that place ... the smells ... the tastes ... the sights ...

... and you can find that my voice starts to work at two levels ... there's a level at which you latch onto my voice ... so whatever I'm saying ... whatever I'm talking about ... just the sound of my voice somehow helps you to relax ... and at the same time ... the ideas and suggestions I give you ... will somehow just flow into the back of your mind ... have a meaning for you ... and you will realise that you can always go back to that special place in your mind ... whenever you feel you want to be calm, secure and relaxed ..."

Arm levitation (based upon a method of Milton Erickson)

Although this method is somewhat time-consuming and does not necessarily lend itself to the majority of dental surgery situations, it is included as an example of the seamless combination of induction and deepening. In addition, the surprising and apparently involuntary levitation of the arm and hand often has a powerful effect of strengthening the patient's confidence in their ability to use hypnosis successfully.

"Now please get yourself comfortable in the chair and just let yourself relax. Bring both your hands down onto your thighs. That's right. Now just keep watching your left hand ... watch it really closely ... and as you do you will notice certain things happening as you relax more and more ... and I'll point these things out to you as they happen ... so now concentrate all your thoughts, all your attention on that left hand ...

Maybe you can focus on the feelings and the sensations in your hand ... perhaps it feels heavy as it rest on your thigh ... feel the texture of the material it rests on against the palm of your hand ... the pressure as your hand rests more and more heavily ... possibly you are aware of tingling sensations in your hand ... spreading to your fingers ... just enjoy these feelings as you relax ...

> *Maybe you have noticed how still and quiet it all is and you possibly begin to wonder when the movement that is there will start show itself ... it will be interesting to see where the movements will first happen ... which of your fingers will start to twitch and move first ... I wonder whether it will be the middle finger, the forefinger, the ring finger or the little finger or even your thumb ... one of the fingers is going to twitch slightly and possibly start to move ... all on its own ... let us concentrate our gaze on your left hand for a moment ... see ... it's starting ... did you notice that finger starting to flicker ... and there's no need to try to make it happen ... no need to try to stop it happening ... but you can just let it happen on its own to as you relax ...*
>
> *That's great! And as you relax even more deeply you possibly become aware as you keep watching your hand that your fingers start to rise a little ... rising away from resting on your thigh ... the feeling that they want to start floating upwards ... as though your fingers and your whole hand is feeling lighter and lighter and seems to want to float upwards more and more ... and you can just let it do that ... no longer pressing heavily onto your thigh ... but starting to grow lighter and lighter ... see that that finger has already raised itself just a little ... and feel that feeling spreading throughout your hand and fingers so that it feels lighter and lighter and is beginning to float upwards slowly into the air. Maybe it feels almost as though there's a balloon on the end of a string tied around your wrist that's tugging and lifting it upwards higher and higher into the air ...*
>
> *And as you keep watching your hand ... and as it rises higher and higher ... maybe you begin to notice that you feel a little tired and a little sleepy ... and you would like to close your eyes ... but please keep them open until I ask you to let them close ... and then when they do you will be able to enjoy this peaceful relaxed feeling to the full ...*
>
> *And now your eyelids are probably getting really heavy and as you watch your hand you notice that your arm is beginning to bend ... and your hand is slowly coming nearer and nearer to your face ... closer and closer, and as that happens your body is a feeling a beautiful feeling of relaxation ... a sense of a drowsiness is flowing through your body and your eyes are starting to blink ... as your hand floats nearer and nearer to your face ... and you keep looking at your hand and can hardly keep your eyes open ... but don't let them close just for a few more moments ... not until your hand lightly brushes against your face ... and as that happens then your eyes close ... your hand drops onto your lap ... and you sink down into the chair deeply, beautifully relaxed ... the most relaxed feeling you have ever known."*

As in any procedure based upon an intrinsic and noticeable physical effect, in this case the arm levitation, it is important that you have an "opt out" position in the event of the phenomenon failing to occur.

If the patient tells you that although the initial tingling feeling has happened the arm just won't rise, you may, with the patient's permission, start the process by gently raising the hand a few inches.

> "*... That's really good ... some people do find this all a little strange at first ... how about if I just gently take your hand* [light grip around the wrist] *and just help it a little to start with* [slowly lifting the hand about 15 cm (12 inches)] *... and as I let go ... it may just stay there briefly on its own ... and then start to float upwards on its own as you become more and more relaxed ...*"

Other patients may find that their hand remains heavy as it rests upon their thigh, and that there is no sense whatever of a change in sensation.

> "*... That's great ... many people find that heaviness is a really useful starting point ... now just allow yourself to relax more and more and as you do so let that heaviness grow until your hand is so heavy that it probably just would not want to move at all ... and now let your eyes close, you sink down into the chair deeply, beautifully relaxed ... the most relaxed feeling you have ever known ...*"

Safeguard

Some patients will enter an apparently deep state of hypnosis extremely quickly and readily. In order to protect all patients, and particularly this group, it is sensible to build certain safeguards into the suggestions you give, generally towards the end of the first session, in effect in the form of post-hypnotic suggestions.

> "*You probably now realise that you have a great ability to use hypnosis, and it's going to be so valuable for you. You'll also find that each time you enter hypnosis it will grow easier and easier for you ... you will enter hypnosis more and more quickly and to a greater and greater depth each time you use it ... and we both know that you will use this ability carefully ... that you will only use hypnosis where it's about helping you in a therapeutic way ... with myself or with another doctor or dentist using it to help you ... and in any other setting ... or if it's in a show or on TV ... it will have no impact on you whatsoever.*"

Summary

There are a virtually infinite number of hypnotic induction techniques, many of which can be learned formally and many of which will develop as part of your experience of using hypnosis. However, initially techniques based upon those described above will allow you to hone your skills and will give a sense of focus to your work as you grow in confidence.

The patient should now be comfortable, with their eyes closed, and you may then move on to deepening this hypnotic experience for them.

8

Deepening

There are many definitions of "hypnosis". Dr Michael Heap defines hypnosis as "... a waking state of awareness (or consciousness), in which a person's attention is detached from his or her immediate environment and is absorbed by inner experiences such as feelings, cognition and imagery"[2], and this is a definition to which we will largely adhere in this book.

From this definition it can be inferred that hypnosis is not an "all or nothing" phenomenon and that the degree of detachment from their environment that the patient experiences will vary not only from individual to individual but even within that same individual from time to time, depending upon a number of considerations. The degree of detachment experienced is popularly known as the *depth* of hypnosis, and there are many formal and informal strategies available by which we might deepen the hypnotic experience for our patients. However, it is important to remain aware that deepening is an integral part of the continuum of a process which includes the build-up of trust and rapport, induction and work carried out upon the patient while in hypnosis, and that the introduction of a deepening strategy should be integrated seamlessly into this process.

In this section we will examine the question of the necessity or otherwise of aiming to achieve depth, the elements influencing the depth of hypnosis that a patient might attain, methods by which deepening may be carried out and appropriate safety measures that must complement deeper states of hypnosis.

There are innumerable procedures described in the literature as "deepening techniques". Some will be described here, but it is quite clear that by their very nature some of the more physically based procedures may not lend themselves readily to the dental situation.

Clinical observation indicates that a motivated individual will achieve the depth of hypnosis that they require at any particular time in order to cope with that particular situation. However, hypnosis might be used in dentistry across an extremely broad spectrum of situations. These may range, for example, from the use of hypnosis in alleviating mild dental anxiety right through to its role as the sole analgesic in the extraction of an impacted lower wisdom tooth. One would correctly assume that the latter would necessitate a greater degree of dissociation than the former. By extension, we might generalise by recognising that the more involved or potentially uncomfortable the dental procedure is likely to be, the greater the depth of hypnosis that is advisable.

It is strongly advised that any procedure demanding a deeper state of hypnosis should include the setting up of an ideomotor signalling response (see Chapter 14). This gives you the means of asking permission and gaining consent before commencing any procedure, at the same time giving the patient a sense of control over the situation, thus protecting both the patient and yourself from misunderstanding and potential trauma.

A clinical observation is that a patient experiencing hypnosis over a protracted period of time is likely spontaneously to experience an increasingly deep state of trance. The corollary to this is that the length of time taken over the alerting process should be proportional to the length of time spent in hypnosis; that is the greater the depth of hypnosis experienced. By this means the patient is given ample time to make the physical and psychological adjustment from dissociation to full awareness in a comfortable manner. Where the deepening procedure has incorporated imagery, suggestions should be made in order to bring the imagery to a pleasant conclusion prior to alerting. The period just prior to the alerting process, and indeed the alerting process itself, is the ideal time for delivering post-hypnotic suggestion and ego-strengthening suggestions (see Chapters 15 and13).

When using any form of suggestion in induction or deepening, it is essential that you are not drawn into a challenging situation by the patient. This is particularly so when using induction or deepening methods tied to physical phenomena. For example, if you were simply to say "your arm is growing heavy" the patient might very well analyse their sensory perceptions and say "no, it's not". You will note from the scripts that follow that suggestions regarding altered states may be given in such a way as to avoid challenges, possibly by incorporating such factors as timing, the degree of physical change, an open approach such as "I wonder if ...", and the use of conditional words such as "perhaps" or "maybe".

Deepening techniques

Progressive relaxation

The term *progressive relaxation* was coined by Edmund Jacobson[3]. Jacobson observed that fatigue and discomfort could result from, and also be increased by, muscle tension. He found that when patients realised the cyclical nature of this relationship they could learn that through progressive relaxation they were able to control their symptoms. Unfortunately Jacobson's method would take between 50 and 200 sessions, obviously making it somewhat unsuitable for the average dental practice.

However, hypnosis allows a gateway into extremely profound relaxation. Following hypnotic induction progressive relaxation can normally be learned and utilised in one session, and by incorporation into a post-hypnotic suggestion the depth of relaxation experienced can be achieved again almost instantaneously at subsequent appointments.

[seamlessly following induction]

"Now ... I'd like you to get as comfortable as you can, and be prepared just to let go ... take a gentle breath ... and as you let the breath out just let everything go ...

... and maybe you can imagine that each time that you breathe out ... with each out-going breath it's like letting your breath out in a deep sigh of relief ... letting go ... and that's all you need to have in your mind ... as you let each breath out it is an internal sigh of relief ...

... Maybe you can imagine how it would feel to let that heavy feeling from your eyelids spread gently to the muscles across your forehead ... around your nose ... around your cheeks ... and around your mouth as you just let everything go ... letting that relaxed feeling flow through all the muscles of your face as you let go ... as the muscles relax and the skin over the muscles feels more and more heavy and smooth as you let any tension just flow away ... as you let go ...

... imagine your jaws relaxing and then let them relax ... so that if your teeth were clenched together let them come just a fraction apart ... and allow your tongue to rest on the floor of your mouth as you let yourself relax even more deeply ...

... and allow that feeling from your jaws to float gently down through your chin and your neck ... and down and right across your shoulders ... just allow your shoulders to relax ... and imagine as your shoulders relax they drop a little and relax easily and effortlessly into a really comfortable position ...

... each breath out is a gentle, comforting sigh of relief as you let everything go ...

... maybe you can imagine that each out-going breath becomes like a wave of relaxation ... and as each breath follows the previous one so each wave of relaxation follows the wave before ... so the relaxation grows deeper and deeper and deeper ...

... and as your shoulders drop, imagine that heavy calm and comfortable feeling flowing easily and gently down your arms ... your upper arms, your forearms, down to your hands and right down to your fingertips ... and you know that you could raise your hands if you wanted to but they're so comfortable, so relaxed, it's easier to let them just rest where they are ... as you let go even more deeply ...

... and as the relaxation soaks through your mind and your body maybe you can almost imagine looking inside yourself ... at your own body ... and if there are any knots of tension anywhere in your mind or your body maybe you can picture crystals gathered in those areas ... crystals of tension ... almost as though you can see the crystals and as you relax maybe you can imagine warm water flowing over the crystals ... just as warm water would dissolve sugar crystals or salt crystals and allow them to flow away ... so the crystals of tension dissolve and flow away and as that happens you become even more relaxed ... sinking down deeper and deeper into the chair ...

> *... deeper and deeper and more deeply relaxed with every outgoing breath ... allowing the feeling to spread through your chest and your stomach ... aware of the slow and steady comfortable calm rhythmic beating of your heart ... aware of the slow calm gentle rhythmic feeling of your breathing as you grow more and more relaxed ...*
>
> *... letting that relaxation spread deeply and more deeply throughout your body ... flowing deeply right through your body ... deeper inside your body right through your body ... down to your legs ... to your thighs ... your knees ... your calves and your ankles and feet ... and right down to your toes ... ... becoming more and more comfortable, calm and relaxed, effortlessly letting go as you allow yourself to relax even more deeply ..."*

Notes

Some practitioners describe progressive relaxation techniques that involve alternate tension and relaxation in order to demonstrate to the patient the difference in feeling between the two. Such a script might include, for example:

> *"... I'd like you to clench your fists as tightly as you can and hold your breath ... and now as you let your breath out allow your hands to unclench and become heavy and very deeply relaxed ..."*

It is our opinion that the technique of alternate suggestions is not generally appropriate when used in hypnosis, primarily because the constant suggesting of tension followed by relaxation may interrupt the natural smooth flow of the process.

Some practitioners prefer to work with a sequence of relaxation that begins at the feet and culminates at the head. We perceive the imagery of relaxation as being of a "melting" nature, and when given the option patients have commented that to them it feels more natural to relax downwards.

Counting

Counting as a form of deepening may be used either as a direct suggestion or in conjunction with appropriate imagery. When using a simple counting deepening technique effectiveness may be greatly increased by coupling it in with the patient's breathing.

First, the patient might be given a simple explanation of what to expect:

> *"... we have a natural reflex ... when we are anxious or surprised we tend to take a gasp of breath ... we tend to hold our breath ... but when the danger's over ... when we let go ... we tend to let our breath out in a sigh of relief ...*
>
> *... so soon I'm going to ask you to hold your breath for just a moment ... and as I say the number ONE I want you to let that breath go ... and as you let go ... to become even more deeply relaxed ... and then we'll do the same again for TWO ... and so on ... and as I say each number, as you let your breath out ... and as you let everything go ... you'll become more and more deeply relaxed ... down into the chair ... OK?"*

Now observe the patient's breathing pattern, and couple the following suggestions in with their natural indrawn breath.

Note that it is not necessary to time this with consecutive breaths, but allow the patient a few seconds of normal breathing between each count.

> *"... now ... if you'd hold your breath for just a moment ... and ONE ... just let that breath out in a sigh of relief as you let everything go ... that's great ... deeper and deeper ... (about 20 seconds of normal breathing) ... and now ... once again ... just hold that breath ... and TWO ... just let that breath out again in a deep sigh of relief as you let everything go ... that's great ... deeper and deeper ... letting yourself relax deeply ... sinking into the chair ...* [continue up to the count of FIVE]"

Counting combined with imagery

Notes

When using imagery in hypnosis it is vital that any image introduced is appropriate to the patient involved, and appropriate to the purpose for which the image is being introduced.

For example many people (particularly those with a tendency to claustrophobia) are disturbed by imagery involving a lift, a person who suffers from hay fever is unlikely to enjoy imagery involving a garden scene, and although lazing on the beach is pleasant for many, there are also those who hate it.

This principle applies similarly to the use of imagery in deepening, and it is wise to let the patient know of the potential imagery to be used and to gain their consent prior to introducing such imagery, and indeed, even before the hypnotic induction.

> *"... it's important that you are happy about the images we're going to be using to help you to become more and more relaxed. For instance, would you be quite happy with the image of yourself in a lift?"* [going down a series of steps, in a garden, on a beach, etc.]

Proceed only when the patient has expressed themselves at ease with your suggestion. Some practitioners will suggest that they are accompanying the patient within their imagery. For example:

"... imagine we are walking together down some steps ..."

We prefer to begin the experience as though accompanying the patient, and then allow the patient to be there on their own within the imagery. For example:

"... imagine that we are on a terrace looking down onto a beautiful garden ... and you decide that you would really like to go down the steps right down into the garden ..."

And then at termination:

"... and you are once again with me on the terrace above that beautiful garden ..."

When introducing images it is important that you set the scene and then the patient is given a "canvas" on which to paint their own image based on the cues they are given. If the description were to be too precise it could easily be at odds with the patient's intuitive vision thereby reducing its efficacy in deepening the hypnotic state. You might aim to emulate Milton Erickson, who is described as being a master of the precise use of vague language[4].

Note in this example the way that this freedom is given to the patient by the use of such words as "perhaps", "maybe", "I wonder if", and note too the multimodality of the suggestions.

[using a garden terrace imagery as a "special place"]

"... I wonder if you can imagine standing with me ... on a terrace looking down onto an absolutely beautiful garden ... maybe it's a garden you recognise from your own store of memories ... or maybe it's somewhere completely new to you ... some people like formal gardens ... and some prefer more informal, natural gardens ... perhaps there are flowers ... a lawn ... paths ... flowers ... maybe ... shrubs ... bushes ... trees ... just gradually let it take shape as you look down from the terrace enjoying the wonderful view and the relaxing feeling it gives you ... the many different colours and hues ... perhaps you can almost smell the flowers ... possibly the feel of a gentle breeze ... maybe the smell of newly cut grass ... perhaps the sounds of birds singing ... it just feels so calm, so peaceful ... so relaxing ...

... and you notice that from our terrace there are five broad steps that take you from the terrace down into the garden ... and the steps are quite shallow and very safe ... there might be handrails ... and you realise how good it would be to walk down the steps ... actually to go down to that beautiful garden ... and so you take a gentle breath ... and as you let it out ... ONE ... you go down the first step ... and you realise that from this angle the garden looks even more beautiful ...

[repeat until the patient is at the garden level]

> *... and now you are so comfortable ... so very, very deeply relaxed ... and you can just let yourself walk around the garden ... enjoying the feeling of the ground beneath your feet ... the perfumes ... the sounds ... how it feels to be in that beautiful garden ... so that for now your mind and body can become totally involved within the garden ... and all the things outside that beautiful image and those lovely feelings just fade away into the background ... as you just enjoy this wonderful feeling of deep relaxation."*

To conclude and before alerting the patient:

> *"... so now it's time for you to leave that garden for the time being ... but you know you can always return to it ...* [here you insert the post-hypnotic suggestion applicable to future appointments] *... so you look around again to impress it all on your memory ... and slowly walk back through the garden the way you came ... and find yourself once more at the steps leading up to the terrace ...* [insert ego-strengthening suggestions] *... and as I count from FIVE to ONE you slowly climb the steps, you realise that gradually you are returning to the real world ... feeling really pleased with yourself ... so relaxed and comfortable ... and now standing with me on that terrace looking out across the garden ... and now slowly opening your eyes again back here with me ..."*

Fractionation

Fractionation involves a repeated series of actions, at each stage of which the patient will become more and more deeply hypnotised. Advantages of this particular method are that it is quick and effective, and that the patient remains in their comfortable position in the dental chair making only minimal physical movements, thus allowing an uninterrupted flow in the progression of deepening.

Note the use of suggestion to reinforce the patient's awareness of the deepening process.

> *"Soon I am going to ask you to open your eyes, but to remain really deeply relaxed throughout your whole body just as you are now ... and then after a few moments I will ask you to close your eyes again and as you do so to become even more relaxed ... you'll probably find that you want to close your eyes before I even ask you to but even though it's hard to keep your eyes open I'd like you to do so until I ask you to close them. OK? ...*
>
> *... So now I'm going to count to three, and at three I'd like you to open your eyes ... one ... two ... three ... (patient opens their eyes) ... and you're probably aware that your eyelids are heavy and you are really so comfortable ... please hold your breath for just a moment ... and as you let that breath out just let your eyelids close and feel yourself relaxing even more deeply ...*

> [after about 20 seconds] ... *and now we're going to repeat that and this time you'll find that your eyelids are so heavy that it may be a struggle to open your eyes ... but please do so ...*
>   [repeat as above] ...
> [after about 20 seconds] ... *and we'll do this one more time ... and this time you may find that your eyelids are so heavy that your eyes just don't want to open ... and if that is the case why not just let them stay closed ...* [patients' eyes may remain closed] ... *so now, once again hold your breath ... and as you let it out just let yourself go so deeply relaxed ... so comfortable ... deeper and deeper ... more deeply relaxed than you'd ever believed possible ..."¥*

Arm levitation followed by heaviness

This method may be used as a continuation of the hand levitation induction described in the previous chapter, or as a deepening technique in its own right.

The patient will be seated in the dental chair with his hands resting comfortably on the armrests. In the dental setting the left hand is preferable to the right for any technique involving physical movement. This is because from the normal seated position of the patient that hand is in your direct sightline, and at the same time allows you clear vision of the patient's face and body so that any other non-verbal cues, such as grimacing or altered breathing pattern, are easily observable.

Suggestions are made that the arm is growing lighter and will rise from the armrest of the chair. When this has taken place further suggestions are made that the arm has become heavy again and will drop back onto the armrest , increasing the depth of relaxation. (It may be helpful at this stage for you gently to guide the arm back into its original position.)

Note that arm heaviness itself may be used as a deepening procedure. The patient is asked to raise their arm quite consciously and hold it steady in the raised position. Suggestions of arm heaviness as described below are then given.

> *"... as you relax with your eyes comfortably closed I'd like you to focus all your attention on the feelings and sensations in your left hand ... almost as though you can see it in your mind's eye as it rests on the armrest ... and then to bring that focus of attention right down to the very fingertips of your hand ... and quite soon you'll start to notice a feeling ... almost like an electrical tingly feeling starting in your fingertips ... and you'll possibly find that tiny flickery movements start to happen in your fingers ... that's great ... and as you relax even more you can start to become even more aware of the feeling of that armrest beneath the palm of your hand as that tingly, flickery feeling grows ...*
>
> *... and perhaps you notice that it's as though your hand is starting to feel lighter and lighter as you relax more and more ... so that soon it starts to rise up ... quite gently*

> and slowly, all of its own accord ... you'll feel it starting to leave the armrest ... just as if you have one of those really light helium balloons attached by a cord to your wrist, and it's tugging your arm upwards higher and higher ... maybe you can even see that happening in your mind's eye ... and of course your arm can bend at the elbow to let your hand start to rise higher and higher ... or maybe it'll rise from your shoulder so that your whole arm becomes lighter and lighter ... higher and higher ... and even more deeply relaxed ...
>
> ... and now you notice that it's as though your hand is being drawn slowly towards your face ... and as that happens and as you relax even more ... soon you'll find that the back of your hand will gently brush against your face ... that's great ...
>
> ... and as that happens you become aware that your hand and arm are starting to feel heavier and heavier ... so heavy ... and as though there's a heavy weight attached to your wrist, your hand and arm start to sink down back down towards the armrest ... and as that happens you relax more and more deeply ... and I'll just guide your hand back to the armrest as it gets so very heavy ... and as it touches the armrest it's almost as though it sinks into the armrest and you just sink into deeper, deeper and deeper relaxation ... and as you relax even more deeply your hand and arm return to normal again and you become even more deeply relaxed."

Arm catalepsy

As in the previous method, the patient is introduced to the concept that physical change or movement may take place without any conscious input, thus there is a positive impact on the patient's perception of the potency of hypnosis. In this example your suggestions are that the patient's arm, when raised, will simply remain in that position until suggestion are given to reverse the effect.

> "... allow your hand and arm to rest on the armrest as you let yourself relax even more ... I'm now gently going to stroke your arm from your shoulder to your wrist ... is that OK? ... [gain the patient's permission either verbally or by ideomotor response]
>
> ... and as I do so you'll be aware that your arm and hand grow lighter and lighter ... as light as a feather ... just as if you have one of those really light helium balloons attached by a cord to your wrist, and it's tugging your arm upwards ... so that if I now help you and take your wrist and lift your arm high up [gently do so] ... it'll just want to stay there on its own ... so that if I let go [do so]
>
> ... it'll just stay there ... comfortably, easily, with no effort whatsoever ... and you can let yourself relax more and more deeply ..."

After a few moments give suggestions to reverse the effect, thus deepening the hypnotic state even more.

> *"... and now, as I speak to you, you can become aware that your hand and arm are starting to feel heavier and heavier ... so heavy ... and as though there's a heavy weight attached to your wrist, your hand and arm start to sink down back down towards the armrest ... and as that happens you relax more and more deeply ... and I'll just guide your hand back to the armrest as it gets so very heavy ... and as it touches the armrest it's almost as though it sinks into the armrest and you just sink into deeper, deeper and deeper relaxation ... and as you relax even more deeply your hand and arm return to normal again and you become even more deeply relaxed ..."*

Deepening by utilising the "hyper-suggestibility" of hypnosis

> *"... as you relax more and more deeply, I am going to help you by calling out numbers as I look at your teeth ... and you'll find that with each number you hear me call out you will relax even more deeply into the chair ... and you'll find you don't even need to listen to the numbers but you'll just be aware of them ... and each number you hear will help you to relax even more ..."*

Here you may begin to chart the patient's teeth, "... lower right eight ...", and so on, and the patient, uncritically accepting the suggestion above, will relax progressively during this procedure.

Deepening by anchors

Physical and verbal anchoring can be an extremely effective form of deepening, always with the proviso that the patient is happy to accept such physical contact.

Following progressive relaxation, place your left hand on the patient's right shoulder with a gentle but firm pressure.

> *"... whenever you feel my hand on your shoulder you will instantly be reminded of how comfortable and relaxed you feel right now ... and that realisation will allow you to become even more relaxed ... so that each time you feel this slight pressure you will feel so calm, comfortable and relaxed ..."*

By use of suitable post-hypnotic suggestions this form of deepening can be used at subsequent appointments as a speedy and effective induction method.

> *"... when you come for your next appointment with me and you are seated in the chair and ready to relax ... you'll feel my hand on your shoulder like it is now ... you will become so very deeply relaxed and calm ... even more so than you are now ..."*

This anchoring may be used in conjunction with a specific agreed word, or the word may simply be used as an anchor in its own right.

> *"... when you come for your next appointment with me and you are seated in the chair and ready to relax ... you'll hear me say the word "calm" and immediately you will become so relaxed and calm ... calm ... even more so than you are now ..."*

Summary

As with induction, there are virtually limitless strategies to produce deepening, and many of these will evolve through your work and individual relationship with each patient. When the patient has learned for themselves that they have the ability to relax deeply in the dental chair, virtually any signal relating to that experience can be used to deepen the hypnotic state.

9

Alerting

The way in which you alert the patient at the end of a session of hypnosis is crucial to the success or otherwise of your intervention. If the alerting procedure is not carried out correctly the patient is likely to feel somewhat confused and disorientated, and this may influence their perception of hypnosis in a negative way.

Alerting should be done gently and smoothly and the patient's return to full awareness must be handled sensitively. In general, the time taken over the alerting process should be proportional to the amount of time that the session has lasted and the depth that you feel the person has experienced.

The alerting process is an ideal time in which to deliver ego-strengthening and post-hypnotic suggestions, obviously tailored to the work done and the future needs of the patient.

"Soon I will be asking you to gently leave hypnosis and return to here and now with me ... knowing that you can use hypnosis again at later times whenever it's suitable to do so ...
... to make it a gradual and pleasant experience for you I will be counting slowly from one to ten, and even though you may feel that you can open your eyes before that I would ask you to keep them closed until I reach the number ten, and then open them ...
so now I'm counting ...

One ... a little lighter

Two ... having really enjoyed and benefited from this session, and ...

Three ... knowing that each time you use hypnosis it will be easier for you ... you will enter hypnosis more and more quickly, more and more deeply ... and with a greater and greater benefit ...

Four ... gradually coming back to here and now ...

Five ... feeling really confident about your ability to use hypnosis in the future ... and so pleased with the way you've handled it today ...

Six ... and so pleased with the way that you have managed your dental treatment ... how comfortable you have felt ... how well you have coped ...

> *Seven ... quite soon I will be asking you to open your eyes ...*
> *Eight ... feeling more and more alert, relaxed yet alert ... increasingly back in touch with where you are here at the dental practice with me ...*
> *Nine ... almost there ... ready to open your eyes ...*
> *And ten ... eyes open ... wide awake ... alert ... ready to get on with your day ..."*

Shorter script

> *"In a few moments I am going to help you to return to full alertness, and when you do come back to full alertness you'll realise how relaxed you have been here at the dentist ... you can be really pleased with the way that you've learned how to relax so well ... and know that you can learn how to return to this deep relaxation even when you are on your own ... so now I'd like you to start to come back to full alertness ... I will be counting slowly from five down to one ... and at each stage you will be growing more and more alert ... and when I reach 'one' you will be wide awake ... alert and yet relaxed ... ready to get on with your day feeling comfortable and wide awake ... five ... four ... three ... two ... one ... eyes open alert and wide awake."*

Inadvertent alerting

There will be times that a patient comes out of hypnosis inadvertently midway through a session of hypnosis or before the alerting procedure has been completed. Here it is advised that you still carry out formal alerting in order to bring the session to a satisfactory conclusion and to dispel any disorientation that the patient might feel.

> *"... are you OK? ... good ... now what I'd like us to do is to bring the session to its natural conclusion ... is that OK? ... good ... so if you would just please close your eyes again for a few moments ... thank you ... and now I'll help you to return to full alertness, and you can be really pleased with the way that you've learned how to relax so well ... and know that you can learn how to return to this deep relaxation even when you are on your own ... so now I'd like you to start to come back to full alertness ... I will be counting slowly down from five down to one ... and at each stage you will be growing more and more alert ... and when I reach 'one' you will be wide awake ... alert and yet relaxed ... ready to get on with your day feeling comfortable and wide awake five ... four ... three ... two ... one ... eyes open alert and wide awake."*

Always gain reassurance from the patient that they feel comfortable and alert, with no "hangover" from the hypnotic session, before they leave the surgery and again before they leave the premises.

10

Hypnotic Communication

Our understanding of a word or a phrase, while obviously depending upon recognition of its literal sense, is also very much dependent upon the way it is delivered and the context within which it is used. The tone, volume and inflection of delivery will influence the listener, as will the context and the facial expression and body language that accompany the verbal message. So this is the point at which the lessons learned earlier in this book regarding environment, rapport, body language and verbal delivery come together to create successful "hypnotic language".

Although scripts may be helpful in the earlier stages, it is important that you feel comfortable with the language you are using. As you relax into your own habitual use of words your presentation will develop quite naturally and effortlessly. At the same time remain aware that rapport can easily be lost if you fail to respect and adapt to the patient's intellect, comprehension and verbal skills. Be flexible but be yourself. Observe the patient closely, watching out for any signs of tension or confusion so that you can adapt and respond to the patient's situation and needs at all times.

Confidence

Act and speak confidently, but at the same time with an air of compassion and understanding. It is important that however you may feel inside, the appearance and attitude presented to the world, and particularly to the nervous patient, is one of quiet confidence and boundless experience. Any hesitancy or uncertainty can give rise to communication barriers and loss of rapport. This inevitably will hinder or even curtail the process of hypnosis. Initially you will probably feel uncertain, and this might well translate into your delivery, particularly if there is a feeling of self-consciousness in using this new technique in front of your nursing staff. For this reason it is sensible to explain thoroughly to practice staff exactly what will be happening, and it is helpful for you to practise hypnosis with willing members of staff, both for their own experience and as a means of perfecting your delivery technique. It may help if you bear in mind that throughout your career as a dentist you have routinely been speaking calmingly to anxious and agitated patients and using hypnosis is simply an extension of that acquired skill.

Occasionally during induction or deepening the patient may giggle possibly through embarrassment or maybe because of the incongruity, as they see it, of their situation. You can ask them if everything is alright, reassure them that this happens quite often, that giggling is a sign that they are fairly relaxed, and that when the giggling has stopped they can let themselves go back to where they were before it started. Again, if the patient indicates that they want to stop the process, or needs to cough or blow their nose, you can reassure them that this is all fine, and then "... now that you've done that, maybe you can close your eyes once again and relax and gently take yourself back to where we were a few moments ago".

Observation

You should constantly monitor the patient for a number of reasons.

- Any physical signs, such as muscles twitching, swallowing or eyes blinking, can be fed back to the patient. For example, "and your eyelids begin to flicker as your eyes feel more and more tired, and you start to feel more relaxed". This encourages the patient to feel that what is happening is exactly what is supposed to happen, and if you comment promptly it can seem as if the blink, twitch or swallow is almost as a result of your suggestion rather than an observation. This will further enhance the hypnosis.

- You will gain an insight into the patient's emotional state. It is important to notice any signs of distress, and to continue reciting suggestions that the patient is becoming more relaxed when they are patently not so doing will obviously seriously undermine the relationship. Other emotions can often be observed and commented on as appropriate.

- You will be able to deliver comments and suggestions of calmness and relaxation more congruently. The body automatically relaxes more when exhaling, and pacing suggestions to the patient's breathing will enhance the effects of suggestions for calm, relaxation and deepening. This technique ties in neatly with the comments above regarding delivery, and allows space for meaningful pauses as the patient inhales.

In this example assume that the significant words are delivered and accentuated in time with the patient's exhalation:

"... *each breath* **out** ... *like a* **sigh** *of relief* ... *feels so* **calm** ... *as you* **relax** ... *more and more* **deeply** ..."

Positives

People will generally respond far better to positive suggestions than to negative suggestions. Certainly, the imagination finds it very difficult, if not impossible, to represent the non-occurrence of an event as a picture. For instance, "a man plants a tree" is very easy to depict, but its opposite, "a man does not plant a tree", is not.

Many of the language characteristics of hypnosis are therefore geared to conceptualising negatives as positives. For example, rather than the negative statement "you will not be anxious", which draws attention to the anxiety, you can say "you will feel more relaxed ... and calm", or to use a valid natural experience, "as you relax you will find yourself becoming so much more calm and comfortable".

In addition there are words that by their very meaning have a negative context. Words such as "pain", "fear" and "hurt" will for the anxious dental patient serve only to augment their existing fears. Similarly the words "needle" or "drill" carry heavy negative connotations.

Using hypnosis within dentistry entails the development of a new vocabulary, which is based almost entirely upon positive language and which eventually becomes the language of all staff working within your dental practice.

There are, however, times where negatives can be used deliberately. An example might be "please don't go into hypnosis just yet". In this case, attention is directed to the idea of hypnosis, at the same time implying the inevitability that hypnosis will happen, and that only the exact time is not certain.

"Trying"

The word "try" generally implies difficulty and probable failure in achieving the required result. It also implies that a degree of effort will be involved in taking the suggested action. For example, saying "try to relax" is giving a very confused and confusing message and is unlikely to help that patient actually to relax.

However, the word "try" can be used effectively in certain contexts. For example, "don't even *try* to listen to my voice" is very effective communication.

Modifying a suggestion

This principle applies when the patient is asked to experience a physiological change such as anaesthesia. Simply suggesting "your hand is getting numb" is presenting the patient with a strange abstract concept that they will possibly *try* to apply consciously. This will generally be far less effective than engaging the imagination and relating the desired effect with a real experience: "... I wonder when you're going to feel a slight tingling sensation in your hand ...".

Verbal delivery

Pace and expression

Phrases should usually be delivered in a calm, unhurried fashion, with pauses when and where necessary. Often, inexperienced operators feel that they must speak continuously, and that if there is the slightest pause then the process will somehow not continue. In fact, with careful preparation and the establishment of sufficient rapport, most patients will be quite happy with pauses. Often the patient will need time to process an idea, and so a pause following a suggestion will aid the hypnotic procedure. For example: "allowing that calm relaxed feeling to spread across your shoulders ... [*pause*] ... so that your shoulders drop ... [*pause*] ... and that same feeling can start to flow gently down your upper arms ...".

Initially you should allow the hypnosis to proceed at the patient's own pace and should obviously never be impatient. However, as the session progresses and more and more suggestions are complied with you will have more freedom within your pace and the manner in which your suggestions are made.

Suggestions are more readily accepted when they are delivered in such a way as to reflect the appropriate emotion. You might subtly act out the words as you use them; for example, the word "relaxation" may be delivered slowly and quietly and drawn out so that each syllable is clearly identifiable. In contrast, when suggesting increased confidence or motivation, and when alerting, your speech should reflect suitable emotions.

Rhythm

Rhythm has long been recognised as a powerful element in bringing about an altered emotional state. Rhythm within hypnotic delivery is similarly an effective way of potentiating the suggestions that you are making, and so your delivery of suggestions should be matched to the patient's natural rhythms as demonstrated, for example, by their breathing and their heart rate.

Repetition

Simply repeating a phrase two or three times, or expressing the idea in a different way, either directly or by using some form of indirect suggestion, can be a very successful device in hypnosis and an effective way of developing a rhythm. Whereas under normal circumstances such repetition could irritate or bore the person, in hypnosis this is not the case, and it will serve to reinforce the suggestions.

For example, "... **deeper** and **deeper** and **deeper** ...more and more **calm** ... more and more **relaxed** ... more and more **comfortable** ..." are phrases that carry their own natural rhythm and readily adapt themselves to coinciding with the patient's outgoing breaths.

Alliteration

Poetry gains much of its impact on the reader or listener by the use of alliteration, defined as "the occurrence of the same letter or sound at the beginning of adjacent or closely connected words" (*OED*). In hypnosis alliteration is a means of emphasising suggestions, while at the same time facilitating a rhythmic delivery. For example: "… gradually feeling more **calm** … more **composed** … more **clearheaded** … as though things are becoming more **crystal clear** … and as a result you are feeling more and more **confident** …".

Assonance
Again a devise used by poets, assonance is defined as "the resemblance of sounds between two syllables in nearby words, arising from the rhyming of two or more accented vowels, but not consonants" (*OED*). For example: "… feel that **soothing movement** as you breathe away so gently …" and "… that **floating** feeling **flowing** through your body …" and "… a **cool, soothing** water spray …". The use of assonance within the rhythm of delivery will potentiate the suggestions being made.

Conjunctions
Rhythm can also be augmented by the use of conjunctions, defined as "word[s] used to connect clauses or sentences or words used in the same clause" (*OED*). Conjunctions play a major role in hypnotic communication. In this context typical conjunctive words include "and", "because", "as", "so".

The use of conjunctions allows you to deliver suggestions in a smooth flow, without the staccato rhythm that would otherwise occur. For example, compare the following scripts: "… the muscles across your forehead can relax … the muscles in your cheeks relax … the muscles around your nose and your mouth can relax …" with "… **as** the muscles across your forehead relax … **so** the muscles in your cheeks relax … **and** the muscles around your nose and your mouth can relax …".

A second value is that by apparently connecting actions you can subtly indicate a cause and effect relationship, thus enhancing the patient's belief in the efficacy of the suggestions. For example: "… **as** you just let your shoulder muscles relax … **so** you notice that feeling flowing down your arms … **and** as that happens maybe your hands are starting to feel heavy …".

Separating the syllables
Rhythm can be established and pace further controlled by breaking multisyllabic words down into their constituent syllables. For example: "allowing that com-fort-able feeling to flow **eff-ort-less-ly** down your upper arms …".

The "yes set"

Socrates proposed that if asking a simple question that would inevitably require an affirmative answer it was likely that subsequent questions would be answered positively. Much more recently Dale Carnegie expanded this technique[5], and it has been used as a "foot in the door" strategy by countless salesmen and saleswomen.

In hypnosis, this technique can be effective with patients who are quite negative, or uncertain. You might ask a series of simple, even mundane questions – "It's cold today, isn't it?" "Your name is Mr Jones?" and so on – before asking more pertinent questions such as "Would you like to learn how to relax more?"

A truism is a statement of fact that people cannot deny. For example, "Can you remember how cold it feels when you put your hand in the snow to make a snowball?" You can direct the patient to nod their head or give an ideomotor response to express their the answer (see Chapter 14). "And after a while, your hands would become more and more numb? ... and can you remember that feeling right now?"

Certain phrases will facilitate a "Yes set". For example: "most people ...", "everyone ...", "you already know how to ...", "sooner or later...".

Authoritarian or permissive, direct and indirect suggestions

Historically, hypnotic suggestions were direct and authoritarian, reflecting what was then the normal relationship between the doctor and the patient. Typically, the hypnotist would have a basic standard induction followed by very direct commands, such as "You are very sleepy" or "When you awaken you will never smoke again". Remember, too, the instruction as given by Professor Bernheim (Chapter 1): "The pain in your head is going to go. It's away! It's gone! You have no more pain!"

To some extent, this inaccurate notion that hypnosis consists of a very profound, sleep-like trance state, followed by immediate and almost miraculous changes, is still fostered today in literature, cinema and the media. Milton Erickson in particular showed that more permissive, indirect communication could be much more effective in many cases.

In modern practice, hypnotic suggestions are given both directly and indirectly. For example, where the direct suggestion might be "your eyelids are so heavy that your eyes will close", a more permissive approach would phrase suggestions in a less commanding way; for example, "... and your eyes can close whenever you are ready to let that happen".

An important point here is that by monitoring the patient's behaviour and background you are able to make suggestions in whatever manner is best suited to that particular patient at that particular time. So the same patient may respond to indirect or direct suggestions given in a permissive or authoritarian manner on different occasions and even within the same session.

In general, an authoritarian approach may be suitable to people who are used to taking orders, and through social conditioning some dental patients may expect this approach from the dentist. Additionally, where a patient has severe toothache or is becoming extremely distressed, a firm, directive approach may be effective. However, many people resent being told what to do, and will respond more favourably if the suggestions take into account that hypnosis is something that they themselves do and not something that the hypnotist forces them to do. If you are perceived as too domineering this can lead to loss of rapport and belief.

A disadvantage of direct suggestions is that if that suggestion is not complied with the patient may begin to lose confidence in their ability to experience hypnosis, and also in the expertise of the therapist. For example, "your hand is beginning to feel lighter and is starting to float upwards" may not be what the patient experiences at that time, whereas "I wonder which hand will start to feel lighter, and how soon that will happen?" does not represent a challenge.

Indirect communication could be said to access the patient's unconscious resources and may involve the patient much more in creating the desired changes. The intention of the communication is not fully understood consciously, and it can stimulate the patient's own resources, letting them feel more responsible for the changes and giving them the sense of being more in control of the situation.

Types of suggestion

The distinctions made below are somewhat artificial in that many suggestions might fit easily into more than one category. The following list is not intended to be a comprehensive one. You are encouraged to study other texts, and above all practise using a variety of suggestions in order to become familiar with different ways of employing them, always tailoring the suggestions to each individual patient.

Implication and questions

The desired effect is assumed or implied, rather than directly suggested. For example: "Would you like to experience hypnosis now or later?" The implication is that the patient will enter hypnosis, and only the exact time is uncertain. Another example would be "I don't know how quickly these changes will occur ...". Again it is implicit that change will occur but the emphasis is placed on the rate at which it will happen.

You must be careful not to convey any doubt in the patient's mind. For example, "Is your hand getting numb?" allows the patient to respond negatively, whereas "I wonder where you will feel the numbness first ... in your fingertips ... or on the back of your hand?" implies that numbness will occur and only its origin is uncertain.

Other examples might be:
"... and will your eyelids start to blink slowly or quickly?"
"... Some people feel very heavy as they become more and more relaxed ... while others may feel as if they are floating ... it will be interesting to note how you experience relaxation."

Covering all possibilities

There is value in a *fail-safe* approach in which *any* response can be taken as the *right* response. Suggestions can be made to cover all types of response. For example:
"... now, it may be your right hand, or it may be your left, that starts to feel lighter ... although with some people it may begin to feel heavier ... and sometimes it may just

remain as it is now ... as you become more and more relaxed ... just noticing carefully what happens ..."

Note the use of the "third person metaphor', a strategy that can convey the suggestion in a totally non-challenging way. For example: "... people have often told me that as they relax more and more deeply they feel a tingling in their finger tips ... maybe that will happen to you ... and if it does, that's fine ... and if it doesn't, that's fine too ..."

It is important that at no time does the patient perceive the suggestion as a challenge and their response, or lack of response, to the suggestion as a failure. This could lead to loss of rapport and confidence in their or your ability, and would hinder the effectiveness of further suggestions.

For instance, if suggestions for hand levitation are having no apparent effect, you might say, "Good, you are obviously in a far deeper state than I thought." This turns a potentially unfavourable response into a success, making further suggestions more likely to be acted upon. You should not give the impression that things are not going well, and at all times should appear confident and comfortable with the way treatment is proceeding.

Embedded suggestions

An embedded suggestion is a form of suggestion incorporated into a longer sentence or story, with the pertinent section emphasised by pauses, altered tone of voice or pace. This conveys the message in a more subtle way, or can give it extra meaning by presenting suggestions in a way that encourages the patient to use those suggestions in their own way. For example: "You may have noticed that when you are feeling relaxed ... your legs feel pleasantly heavy" or "Let me explain a little bit about hypnosis ... and what you are likely to experience when you go into your own hypnotic state ..."

Linking suggestions

This involves linking the suggestion to previous undeniable statements, and although there may be no logical connection, through linkage the suggestion is more likely to be effective. For example: "You know what it is like to feel the wind on your face, and to see the sun rise ... and you know what it is like to hear the birds singing in the morning ... and because you have all these experiences you will be able to use self-hypnosis very effectively ..." or "... and as you breathe out, so your body lets go of any remaining tension ...".

Illusion of choice

This can be an effective technique that appears to give the patient many choices, but where all the choices will lead to the desired effect. For example: "You can allow your body to relax from your toes up to your head, or you may prefer to let the relaxation flow down from your head to your toes, or maybe you can just let your body relax in whatever way seems best for it."

A *double bind* occurs when the options are not as obvious consciously.

"What is really interesting is that the conscious part of your mind may or may not be aware of these important changes that you have made today."

Or:

"Do you want to go into hypnosis with your spectacles on or off?"

Table 10.1 **Summary of the use of suggestion**

Summary of the use of suggestion	
Establish rapport and cooperative relationship	*Create positive expectancy* (being confident that the suggestion works)
Law of reversed effect (the harder one consciously endeavours to do something, the more difficult it becomes to succeed)	*Law of concentrated attention; repetition of a suggestion* (several – i.e. three or four – times)
The principle of the success of approximation (allow time for the development of the response, don't expect immediate results: e.g. "soon you'll sense a lightness starting to develop in that hand … you can begin to wonder just when you'll first sense a sensation of movement … and that hand is becoming lighter")	*The principle of positive wording of suggestion* (instead of saying "you won't eat sweets too much" you may suggest, "you will protect your body, treating it with kindness and respect")
The carrot principle (instead of pushing people from behind, motivate them from in front, towards a goal, e.g. "you're going to feel so good")	*Law of dominant effect* Stir the emotions of the patient and connect suggestions to them)
The principle of positive reinforcement (giving verbal and/or non-verbal reinforcement: "good", "uhumm", etc.)	*Creating an acceptance or "Yes set"* (using truisms, undeniable statements of fact, makes it difficult for the patient not to continue responding affirmatively to the suggestions that follow)
The principle of interspersing and embedding suggestions (within stories, anecdotes, tales)	*The principle of utilising the patient's cues* (language patterns, non-verbal behaviour)
Principle of confirming the acceptability of suggestions (obtain any kind of commitment that will increase the likelihood of accepting subsequent ideas)	*Principle of a visualisation of the desired effect* (a visual image of the desired effect makes suggestions more potent: "just visualise how fabulous your smile is going to look")
Use proper style/type of suggestion (permissive or commanding, direct or indirect)	*Use the word do, rather than try* (trying implies doubt: "try to raise your hand")

Based on Hammond DC, Hypnotic suggestions and metaphors. New York: Norton & Co., 1991.

11

Ericksonian Suggestions

Milton H. Erickson is a major influence in the field of hypnosis and even now the "Ericksonian Approach", a label that Erickson himself refuted, is widely used. Erickson insisted that he dealt with each person individually using whatever methods seemed appropriate at that time, and that there was no such thing as the "Ericksonian Approach". He was idiosyncratic and ahead of his time in many ways and was often misunderstood by his peers, but the libraries of books testifying to his skills and personality are a measure of his massive influence in modern hypnotic thought.

Although there has been considerable emphasis on Erickson's use of stories and metaphors and his use of indirect, permissive techniques, he would in fact often use direct suggestions and could be very authoritarian when he felt it was necessary.

A great attribute was his exceptional power of observation. He was able to discern many aspects of the patient such as skin tone and body language and aspects of unconscious and conscious behaviour, and to use those observations extremely effectively in formulating a treatment plan, as well as in carrying out treatment itself. He was extremely flexible and unorthodox, related easily to people, and had a great sense of humour. These qualities helped to make Erickson such a formidable therapist, and are very useful attributes for any therapist to cultivate.

In spite of Erickson's reluctance to categorise his work, a number of the techniques discussed throughout this book can be attributed to his influence.

One of Erickson's fundamental beliefs was that everyone has within them the potential resources to solve all their problems, but these resources are often not readily available. He would describe them as being in the unconscious mind. He felt that the role of the therapist was to guide the patient towards these unconscious resources so that the patient could then resolve their problems. Consequently, he did not consider investigating and discovering the causes of the patient's problems to be necessarily important, but focused on how best to bring out the patient's own strengths and abilities. At a time when psychiatry and hypnosis were centred around the psychodynamics of illness, this was considered a highly radical approach. The following descriptions are of some of the techniques of suggestion employed by Erickson. Others are described elsewhere in the text.

Symptom prescription

The patient is invited to intensify their problem or even cause the problem to become worse. For example, you may ask the patient to increase the intensity of their pain or the strength of their anxious feelings. When the patient has achieved this you can point out to them that they have actually exercised some control over something that previously they felt was uncontrollable. If they can cause that feeling or behaviour to change for the worse, they must be able to change it for the better.

> *"Sometimes people tell me that even thinking about the pain can make it worse ... ? I wonder if you can imagine how it would feel if it were worse right now ... just go back to some time when it was really bad ... maybe you can imagine the pain on a scale of 0 to 10 ... see if you can take it up by a point ... whether you can make it just a little worse just now? ...*
>
> [get affirmation]
>
> *... so now we can see that your thoughts and imagination can alter that pain ... isn't that fantastic ... you can actually control that pain by your imagination ...*
>
> *Now wouldn't it be great if we could train your imagination ... would you like me to show you how you can use your own imagination to help to move it in the other direction ... to let that pain you had fade away ... to help you to feel better? ... maybe even just a little bit at a time ..."*

Open-ended questions

Therapists, as well as patients, do not always know the best way to proceed with treatment. Erickson felt that a certain form of open-ended question would allow the patient's unconscious to select the best therapeutic response.

One patient sought help to stop smoking after stopping on two previous occasions, once for nine months, and once for three months. Each time, she started again when faced with very stressful events. This lady was capable of giving up smoking, she was highly motivated and she was convinced that hypnosis would enable her to stop again. The techniques as described in the chapter on smoking cessation were used, together with the following:

> *"We all have potentials that we are unaware of, and we do not usually know how they will be expressed. Now that you have finally set yourself free, I wonder, just how will your inner mind choose to deal with any future crises?"*

Not knowing, not doing

Erickson would make suggestions in this way in order to induce changes that seemed to occur by themselves, without any apparent effort from the patient. When a patient is relaxed, as is usually the case in hypnosis, he is predisposed *not to do*, rather than *to do* something, and we *do not know* how the unconscious part of our mind is functioning. *Not knowing* and *not doing* emphasise the automatic nature of hypnosis, which can be useful for some patients. For example:

"You do not even need to keep your eyes open."

"You do not have to listen to me because your unconscious mind can do that and respond all by itself."

Utilisation

This term was used by Erickson to convey a complete acceptance of whatever happened, so that whatever the patient did or said could be used, in one way or another.

For example, upon noticing a patient yawn, Erickson said: "Have you ever noticed how after a yawn, your whole body relaxes more deeply?"

If a patient believed that they were stubborn he would take that as a very positive trait, and congratulate them: "Great! That's just what is needed in this situation, you need to be stubborn to persist in giving up smoking!"

Negatives

Erickson observed that some people resented being over-directed, or even being directed at all, and they would resist suggestions or even do the opposite in order to negate the suggestion. By using phrases such as the following he would defuse their resistance or inhibitions[6].

"You can try, can't you?"

"You will, will you not?"

"Why not let that happen?"

Interspersal suggestions

Erickson would utilise this technique frequently, using metaphors and stories taken from the patient's experiences, his own experiences, other people's experiences or from life and nature in general[7].

An Ericksonian induction by means of embedded suggestion

"Let me tell you a little about hypnosis, and what you **may well experience in hypnosis.** *Hypnosis comes from the Greek word 'hypnos' meaning sleep. Now the reason it is called hypnosis is not because people actually are asleep, but can look as if they are to others. This is because you are sitting or lying with* **your eyes comfortably closed,** *all your body* gently relaxing *... your mind* remaining alert ... and focused ... *just your body* gently relaxing.

So, you can recognise that hypnosis is a natural state of body and mind ... that you have experienced many times ... and perhaps you can remember a time *when you were waking up one morning, with no need to rush, and as you lay there with a growing* inner feeling of comfort *... there may have been times when you were* forgetting about your body *... resting comfortably ... and as you lay there,* gently drifting *... as if dreaming ... and then later waking* surprised at how much time has gone by.

Or there may well have been times when you have sat down in a comfortable chair with a good book, and although at first you are very aware of all the sound around you, you gradually become so absorbed in the images that arise ... more and more absorbed in that inner world you have created ... *that you can become* unaware of everything going on around you. *Often, as you continue to read,* feeling warm, comfortable and relaxed *... you find your* eyes begin to feel tired ... *and no matter* how hard you try to keep your eyes open ... they just feel more and more tired .... And your eyelids feel heavy ... *until* ... your eyes gently close .... *This is what most people experience in hypnosis,* feeling comfortably relaxed ... . Letting the eyes close naturally ... . Feeling more and more relaxed with each breath ... *And some people* notice the thoughts becoming more and more clear, and lucid ... *whereas others* recall pleasant memories, past successes .... *Or maybe* look forward to something ... relaxing without any conscious effort ... more and more absorbed in the experiences.

And even when very deeply relaxed ... you know that one part of your mind is watching out ... and so you know you are safe ... and this allows you to become even more deeply relaxed.

So, now you know that you have been experiencing hypnosis, in a way, all of your life, and you can feel safe *in the knowledge that you* already know how to go into hypnosis ... in your own special way."

Metaphors and images are used extensively in hypnosis to potentiate suggestions, and this topic is the subject of the next chapter.

12

The Use of Metaphor

Throughout history, be it in the writings of Homer, Aesop or the Bible, wide-ranging lessons and moral teachings have been communicated by metaphors integrated within stories. Typically the story will present someone or something (for example, an animal) that is troubled and searching for a way out of their problem. The story will describe a series of obstacles that will need to be overcome until ultimately, with or without help from an external agency, the hero will usually find a solution and emerge triumphant and happy.

In more modern times we see a similar use of storytelling, for example in the tales of the Brothers Grimm and Hans Christian Andersen, and the ensuing films of Walt Disney, where the handsome young prince must overcome death-defying odds and fiendish challenges in order to claim the beautiful princess imprisoned within a seemingly impregnable castle. The imagination and emotions of the reader/cinema-goer become totally engaged, so that for instance even though in the film *ET* the more insightful members of the audience were aware that the creature was an electronic model, the many tears shed at ET's predicaments, loneliness and ultimate departure were genuine.

So we can see that the purpose of the story is that the reader/listener will be drawn in emotionally and will identify with the problems and persona of the hero, and through the symbolism of the story find a pathway to solutions of his own problems. In other words the story with its characters and predicaments becomes a *metaphor* for the recipient.

Within the stories there are *symbols* – beings, objects, obstacles and situations that represent something else, for example the high wall that must be climbed or the stormy sea voyage that must be navigated in order to gain the prize.

A metaphor is defined as "the application of a name or descriptive term or phrase to which it is imaginatively, but not literally, applicable" (*OED*). So it is important always to remember that the metaphor is not an exact description of a situation. Rather it is a representation of how that person perceives the situation to be at that time – a description of their world. Similarly your understanding and mental acceptance of the metaphor is a representation of the world as *you* see it at that time. If you handle a patient's metaphor inappropriately, for example by forcing your own interpretation back onto the patient, a damaging lack of mutual understanding can arise. As a professional your role should become more reflective, reflecting back your interpretation in such a way as to gain clarification and resolution:

"... so you feel that this surgery is like a torture chamber ... that must be awful for you ... maybe you can tell me what it is exactly that gives you that feeling? ..."

The metaphor in written words

Possibly the most widely used form of metaphor is in the written word. Why should the letters "RED" give us a visual image of a colour and the letters "CAR" generate the image of a vehicle? In fact almost every word we use is representative of a subjective image that the reader or listener will interpret in his own subjective way and integrate into his own world.

The mechanism by which this works is known as *transderivational search*, the internal equivalent of the "Google search" we might carry out on our computer; an almost instantaneous cross-referencing of all the information and background at our disposal in order to make sense of the letters. And it is this transderivational search, this *unconscious* inner probing, that creates the power of the metaphor.

Our general use of metaphors

We employ symbols and metaphors commonly in normal conversation, and although their use is seemingly at an unconscious level, they are generally clearly understood by the receiver. In fact it is the hidden communication of metaphor that gives it much of its potential for bringing about change in the recipient. Additionally, one or two words of metaphor can be used to create a complex picture, which despite its complexity is readily interpreted and understood.

"We've got a mountain to climb."
"Keep your hat on!"
"Don't get your knickers in a twist!"

Proverbs also are widely used to express a message in easily understood metaphorical ways. To someone who seems to be taking success for granted we might say "Don't count your chickens before they're hatched", and a common piece of advice for individuals who spend time regretting past events is "It's no use crying over spilt milk". What is of overriding importance here is the care that must be taken over the appropriateness or otherwise of that metaphor to that person at that time. An inappropriately delivered metaphor or proverb can seem patronising and can create anger and dismissal within the recipient.

Patients will often use metaphors, particularly in attempting to describe pain:

"It's a stabbing pain ... it goes through me like a knife."
"It's like being kicked by a horse."
"It's a shooting pain."

A common aggravating feature of pain is that the patient will often feel that the pain is beyond their control and thus unmanageable. Metaphor can be used to give the pain colour, physical size, weight, temperature, shape and texture so that the patient can devise ways of modifying and lessening their pain (see Chapter 25).

So metaphors incorporate things that are familiar to us to explain things that are less so. They can convert abstractions into images to which people can respond more readily. As the saying goes, "a picture paints a thousand words". The mental imagery produced makes the communication far more effective.

Metaphors can be used to illustrate key points, to encourage self-reflection, to increase motivation and to help patients to reframe thoughts and attitudes. The powerful impact of a metaphor helps us to remember, providing information on more than one level and facilitating new patterns of thought.

Metaphors can be used to encourage the patient to put their own interpretation on a message, which consequently involves them more actively in the therapy.

Hypnosis and metaphor

If metaphor is used so generally and effectively in conversation, what is it that makes hypnosis such a good vehicle for the use of metaphor and storytelling? After all, in earlier sections we have examined very effective directive and less directive ways both of inducing hypnosis and employing hypnotic suggestions.

An answer is that among the qualities of the mind set that we call hypnosis there is increased acceptance of suggestion, with corresponding reduction in critical analysis and immersion in the world of the hypnotic fantasy. All of these factors will combine to reduce the patient's judgement and rationalisation of the metaphor, allowing largely uninhibited acceptance of the metaphor and generation of a relevant meaning and value in therapy.

Metaphor in hypnosis makes use of the application of *indirect suggestion*, an approach much used by Milton Erickson.

Metaphors in ego-strengthening and de-stressing

Although the ego-strengthening suggestions you give patients will often be fairly specific and related to the actual treatment and the performance of the patients concerned ("... feeling so much more calm ... more confident ... so pleased with what you've achieved ..."), the use of metaphors can create a more subtle and extremely effective form of suggestion. It is particularly important that the metaphor you use relates to that patient as an individual, and so gleaning a fragment of knowledge of the patient's background is invaluable.

> For example, if that patient is at all interested in gardening:
> *"I know that you're aware ... that when you plant a seed in the rich, fertile ground ... you make sure it has enough water to sustain and nourish it ... but otherwise, you allow it to develop ... without interference ... trusting that the seed will bloom and flourish ... in its own good time ... just like the suggestions planted in your unconscious mind today."*

Note that within this metaphor there is no reference to the actual therapy involved, allowing the patient to make their own connections and interpretations.

> This further example might be used with a person involved with music:
> *"... you might know as well as anyone ... that whenever violinists have finished playing ... they will loosen the strings ... gently ... gradually ... to allow the tension to release ... to make sure that the instrument remains in perfect condition ... stress-free ... I guess you could even say ... healthy ..."*

Extended metaphors in storytelling

This leads us quite naturally into the extended metaphor, characterised by storytelling. This subject will be looked at in more detail in relation to hypnosis in children's dentistry (see Chapter 31), but storytelling can also be used effectively with many adults.

The storyteller has been an important part of social history from very earliest records of human development. As until quite recent history few people could read, they would gather around the storyteller or the wandering minstrel. Entranced by the devices of oratory – rhythm, animation, characterisation, variety in the tone, pitch and volume of voice – the listener would become focused and absorbed in the story at the expense of their contact with the outside world – a state much akin to hypnosis. So the act of telling a story, if done well, can be "hypnotic". You can induce hypnosis by the storytelling and use it at one time for both deepening the trance state and for carrying out therapy.

Conversely, making the story as boring as possible, speaking slowly, in a droning, monotonous voice about tedious everyday things, can also induce a trance, as the recipient attempts to escape from the boredom. We have probably all experienced this in conversation with certain acquaintances, but it can also have a therapeutic application, as Erickson often demonstrated.

"Other person" metaphor

Stories allow you to introduce ideas indirectly in order to engage the patient's own resources, so a story will be more acceptable if it relates in some way to that patient's circumstances. A particularly effective use of metaphor might be seen in the use of the "other person" strategy in which you can attach the patient's problem to another patient (without divulging any personal details). It is generally more effective to tell the story and then move on without any analysis, allowing the patient to integrate the meaning "unconsciously".

> "... it's strange because as you were telling me about your problem I remembered some-one I saw a few years ago ... [here sketch in rough description of the other person, giving similarities so that the patient can identify with them] ... and they found that hypnosis worked really well ... and when I saw them again recently they were look-ing so good and seemed so much more confident ..."

An extension of this might be to use *yourself* as the metaphorical other person. Milton Erickson would utilise embedded suggestions frequently, using metaphors and stories taken from the patient's experiences, his own experiences, other people's experiences or from life in general[8]. An example is of Erickson's telling a man suffering from tinnitus of how he once spent a night in a factory and learned naturally to block out the noise of the machinery[9].

Imagery

The power of metaphors and stories is their role in the creation of images within the recipient's mind. When we use the term "imagery" within the framework of hypnosis we refer not only to visual imagery, but to a fusion of mental pictures, sounds, tastes and smells, as well as such physical factors as temperature, weight and texture, and also the inner feelings within the person's body.

All of us use imagery virtually all the time we are awake, and in dreams when we are asleep. The relation of the reality around us and the imagery it spontaneously creates for us is our way of positioning ourselves within our world. It is part of what makes us human. We use imagery to solve problems and to recreate emotions, sensory experiences and memories.

We plan for the future through imagery. A sports psychologist will use the visualisa-tion and accompanying feeling and emotions of winning a race to prime an athlete, and in health care forward pacing, encouraging a person to visualise themselves looking and feeling good at some future time, might be used as an aid to weight reduction and habit management and, of course, dentistry.

A brief exercise

- Please concentrate on this word ...
- "BOAT".
- And once again say to yourself very slowly ... "BOAT".
- Then please sit back, and close your eyes for about 10 to 15 seconds.
- Now let's examine what just happened.
- And remember that you were not asked to *think* about a boat or even to *imagine* one, but simply to read the word on the page.
- When you closed your eyes you probably created a spontaneous image of a boat.
- No one else can have any idea of what image may have appeared in your mind and what your particular boat looked like.
- Possibly you didn't get a visual image at all, but just a feeling associated with the word.
- If a visual image did float into your head, maybe it was of a sailing boat, maybe a cruiser, maybe a child's drawing of a boat, maybe a yacht, maybe a toy boat.
- Maybe the particular boat that sailed through your mind had to do with something in your life like a holiday or a boat trip that you'd taken years ago. Or maybe not.
- Perhaps the image that came to you upset you. Although "boat" is a relatively neutral word, for some people it may have upsetting connotations relating, for example, to accidents or seasickness.

The sequence of events:

1. You saw and read a random, fairly neutral word.
2. When you closed your eyes (or maybe even before then), almost by reflex an image representing that word floated through your mind. (Note that this would have happened, possibly more powerfully, if you had heard the word spoken.)
3. Again almost by reflex, the image triggered off recall of an associated experience.
4. And this in turn triggered off an emotional response ... if the recall was of a wonderful holiday in the sun you possibly felt happy and relaxed, but perhaps this image triggered a less pleasant effect.
5. When we are agitated or tense we release adrenalin-related hormones to a much greater extent than when we are relaxed.
6. *So that simple word possibly had a profound effect on your body's hormonal system.*

And all of this happened within a brief instant of time.

So to summarise, we can say that for most of us any word we hear or see, or indeed any sensory input, carries within it a suggestion that is totally individual to the recipient of that sensory input.

And the image will generally trigger off one or a number of emotions, which in turn will affect the way that individual feels.

And through conditioning, that feeling will conjure up further associations, further images and further feelings.

Unfortunately, we all too frequently allow this process to work against our best interests. Certain procedures, for example a visit to the dentist, will for many people automatically conjure up unpleasant, fearful images, causing varying degrees of anxiety. And this in turn will give rise to further associated imagery with an ensuing physiological response, heightening those emotions.

So someone who imagines an unpleasant dental experience, remembers a previous visit or anticipates an appointment to come, feels anxious or frightened, and can experience physical discomfort such as increased heart rate and all the other signs of autonomic arousal merely from the mental images.

However, the positive side of this is that imagery can be one of the tools we use in hypnosis to help influence the way people think, feel and act, in order to promote constructive change.

Sensory modes

Visual imagery is the primary, but not the only, representational sense of most people. We all take in, process and impart information slightly differently from one another. Other senses involved might be visual, auditory, kinaesthetic (relating to physical feelings), olfactory or gustatory. For most people visual imagery dominates but the most effective imagery will involve more than one sense, and with practice it is possible to improve one's ability to use all of these senses.

In setting up visualisation you should encourage the patient to use all the senses that may be related; for example, to see the event in colour, in motion, cold or hot, wet or dry. Some patients can have a sense of their body moving in relation to their surroundings, or can experience fatigue or a feeling of energy. It is important to note these internal feelings such as a sense of achievement, satisfaction or sadness.

The patient's own imagery is always to be preferred, and it is important that you are not drawn into using your own, although you might be prepared to prompt if there is an obvious block. It is important, too, to reassure the patient that whatever images surface, they are acceptable and relevant. In this way the patient will not feel as though their imagery is not working or they are doing it wrongly. Not everyone will get explicit, intense images, especially to begin with, and encouragement may be necessary to prevent a sense of failure.

Uses of imagery

"Special place"
Here you may invite the patient to imagine a place where they feel totally relaxed, totally at ease, safe and secure, calm and peaceful. Suggest that whenever the patient visits this haven these feelings can become intensified. Generally this will be an imaginary

place constructed by the patient with your help, that they can return to again and again at their times of need. The special place can be inside or outdoors, it can be somewhere that they have been, or would like to go to, or it could be a place that is a complete fantasy.

It is important not to allow your own imagery to intrude upon this scene – it belongs to the patient. This means that your input must be general, but always directed towards the specific needs. Do not use the word "think", but encourage the patient to "be there", letting images "float in and out of your mind".

If the patient cannot bring an appropriate image to mind, you may have to take the initiative, but be careful not to be too specific, and firstly ask a few questions to determine that person's preferences. Do not, for example take them to a beach unless they like beaches or to the countryside if they are hay-fever sufferers. Let the patient know of the potential imagery to be used and to gain their consent prior to introducing such imagery, and indeed, even before the hypnotic induction. Proceed only when the patient has expressed themselves at ease with your suggestion.

In setting up the image in hypnosis the patient can be given freedom by the use of alternatives:

> *"... it may be a memory of somewhere long ago ... or perhaps it's really recent ... may even be fantasy ... and it doesn't matter which ... it may be indoors or outside ... some people relax by doing very little and others find they relax with activity ... it really doesn't matter ... maybe alone ... maybe with others ... maybe it's so real you can almost feel it ... the sounds ... the smells ... and seeing the colours ... feeling how good it feels ..."*

Habit control and "forward pacing"

Imagery can be used to great effect in the management of smoking cessation and other forms of habit correction (see Chapter 26). For a smoker the image might take the form of some time in the future when they have become a non-smoker. They might then be helped to generate an image of themselves as a non-smoker, experiencing themselves living a full, happy life in the absence of tobacco.

For others the imagery may be of themselves with straight, healthy teeth when they have had their orthodontic treatment, or when they no longer suck their thumb or bite their fingernails. In this way the imagery is depicting the patient's success rather than the negativity that they perceive in maintaining the habit – a carrot rather than a stick.

Relaxation

Imagery can be used directly to reduce physical and psychological tension. Firstly invite the patient to describe their perception of the tension and listen carefully to the metaphors and images they use. Commonly tension is described as, for example, "wound up like a spring" or "like tightly stretched wire". With the patient in hypnosis, use your own imagination to relieve the tension, constantly using the imagery with which the patient has presented you.

Pain control

Imagery is an extremely effective adjunct to hypnotic pain management, and this is described in detail in Chapter 25.

References

1. Elman D. Hypnotherapy. Glendale, CA: Westwood Publishing Co, 1977.
2. Heap M. A definition of hypnosis. In: Hypnosis. Sheffield: University of Sheffield, 1990.
3. Jacobson E. Progressive Relaxation. Chicago: University of Chicago Press, 1938.
4. Battino R. Guided Imagery and Other Approaches to Healing. Carmarthen: Crown House Publishing, 2000.
5. Carnegie D. How to Make Friends and Influence People. New York: Pocket Books, 1990.
6. Erickson M, Rossi E. Hypnotic Realities: The Induction of Clinical Hypnosis and Forms of Indirect Suggestion. New York: Irvington, 1976.
7. Erickson M. The interspersal hypnotic technique for symptom correction and pain control. Am J Clin Hypn 1966;8:198-209.
8. Erickson M, Rossi E. Hypnotherapy: An Exploratory Casebook. New York: Irvington, 1979.
9. Gordon D. Therapeutic Metaphors. Cupertino, NY: Meta Publications, 1978.

Ego-strengthening

"Every day, in every way, I am getting better and better." These words of Emile Coué[1], the noted French psychologist, are often quoted among those seeking self-improvement. If you are feeling particularly low in self-esteem the words can have a hollow ring, but in the absence of self-criticism they can have the potential of inspiring great change. Hypnosis is characterised by a greatly reduced critical faculty; suggestions are not subject to the degree of analysis that we usually employ. Consequently hypnosis is a potent facilitator of what has come to be known as *ego-strengthening*. In short, ego-strengthening in hypnosis comes as the effect of virtually anything you say or do that enhances the patient's self-esteem and self-confidence.

The concept of ego-strengthening in hypnosis is generally credited to John Hartland, and is explained and illustrated at length in his book *Medical and Dental Hypnosis and its Clinical Applications*[2]. His original script has been used and modified by generations of doctors and dentists, and Hartland himself felt that it was an essential part of every treatment, and in many cases was the main reason for their success. Although the scripts devised by Hartland may now seem somewhat outdated and authoritarian, they lend themselves readily to modification and can serve as a useful template for the student of clinical hypnosis.

The purposes of ego-strengthening are to increase the patient's confidence and self-belief, to make them aware of their ability to cope and to increase their sense of self-reliance. As a result the patient can develop a sense of control of their situation leading to a reduction in their anxiety and worry.

All of these factors can be very useful in helping patients to cope with dental treatment and in facilitating each successive aspect of the treatment, as well in encouraging improvements in patients' dental and oral health.

Timing and tone of suggestions

As many people will respond negatively to suggestions that they perceive as being unrealistic, an important factor of ego-strengthening is its timing. For example, simply telling a nervous patient that they will feel more in control might sound unbelievable and could lead to their losing confidence in your judgement. Initially there must be rapport so that the patient can feel confident in their relationship with you and optimistic about their treatment. Ego-strengthening suggestions should be directed specifically toward that particular patient's needs, and delivered in a way that is best suited to them. Very often the suggestions may be based upon feeding back to the patient the success of an action they have just carried out:

> *"... that's terrific ... just feel how good it is to know that you've sat still with your mouth open for me to examine all your teeth ... even though when you first came you didn't think it would be possible ... and now you can use that feeling of confidence to take your treatment a bit further ..."*

The Ego

The concept of the Ego is based on the psychoanalytical writings of Sigmund Freud[3], but over the years since then the word has come into much more general usage in a variety of contexts. Freud postulated that each human being has within his personality three main components, respectively the *Id*, the *Ego* and the *Superego*, and that these attributes cause us to behave as we do and also define us as individuals.

He regarded the Ego as representing and enforcing the *reality principle*, in contrast to the uncoordinated instinctual Id, which is concerned only with the *pleasure principle*. An example of the workings of the Id may be drawn from the experience of a hungry baby. During feeding the infant sees, smells, touches and tastes food, and these experiences are stored in memory as the linkage between food and pleasure. If in future the infant's hunger is not satisfied, images are formed in the mind in an attempt to achieve gratification but are obviously unsuccessful, thereby creating tension. In response the infant develops ways of communicating within the real world in order to relieve this tension, and begins to react and respond within his environment. Freud named this objective part of the personality the Ego, and saw it as the individual's quest to hold the subjective Id in check by asking itself: "Is there a means of alleviating this tension? How do I acquire it?"

Freud saw the Ego as a defence against the Superego, the attribute that seeks to control what it deems unacceptable desires, and which contains our conscience. The Superego is the part of our mind that knows what is right or wrong according to the rules of the society in which we live and that causes us to feel guilt when we think or do something wrong, and pleasure when we think or do something right.

Freud has represented the Ego as continually struggling to defend itself from three dangers or masters: "from the external world, from the libido of the Id, and from the severity of the Super-ego"[3].

In the modern context the word "ego" is widely used. We speak of someone as having a "massive ego", being an "egomaniac" and as being "egotistical". We refer to a hidden part of ourselves as our "alter-ego", and describe someone who is overly meek and reluctant to express their opinion as having a "lack of ego" or a "deflated ego". All of this indicates that an individual's ego can grow or shrink, or can become strengthened or weakened by their perception of their environment at any particular time.

In dentistry

So we can understand how at a visit to the dentist the internal and external pressures perceived by an anxious or fearful patient can contribute to a greatly reduced and weakened ego state. The patient's Id will be urging them to run away and their Superego will be attempting to control their behaviour and to do "the right thing" by having their teeth treated. In the middle of this sandwich is their Ego which is being pulled, pushed and squashed in all directions, and considerably weakened by these tensions.

The patient will characteristically be in a state of lowered self-esteem when attending for dental treatment. Often patients will express their guilt and shame: "I'm a terrible patient. I'm so scared. I bet I'm the worst patient you've ever seen. I've not been to the dentist for so long I'm ashamed to let you look at my teeth." Often there may be regression to an almost childlike state of dependency, not infrequently accompanied by sobbing and other aspects of childlike behaviour.

The concept of self-efficacy has become widely accepted as important in enabling people to overcome problems and to maintain in later life the improvements made within therapy. Ego-strengthening is a major tool in guiding the nervous dental patient from their initial state of dependency into a state of adult autonomy. The increased suggestibility and enhanced imagery that characterise hypnosis make the medium particularly valuable in facilitating ego-strengthening, and it is possible to find a use for ego-strengthening in virtually every aspect of dental treatment.

Although ego-strengthening may largely be by complimenting and thereby reinforcing, it is important that this is not done in a patronising way as this could damage the dentist–patient relationship. It should always be appreciated that as small as each forward step made by the patient may seem, to that patient it may represent a great forward leap. Reassuring the patient that many people share the problem of dental fear, and congratulating them on having made the decision to make and keep their appointment, can feed back a success orientation. Emphasising that dental treatment is a *team* task – "... now you're here we can really work together to sort out your problem ..." – can help the patient to progress from childlike dependency into an adult relationship.

Ego-strengthening might consist of the insertion of short phrases, such as:

> *"You may be surprised how easily and how quickly you become deeply relaxed the next time you experience hypnosis."*

111

> *"That's terrific … you must be quite thrilled at how well you managed that … You have shown today that you can start to control your thoughts, and so your feelings, and consequently even your behaviour. I wonder just how quickly this control will increase as the days go by?"*

Ego-strengthening (after J. Hartland)

In reading the following you will be aware of its, by modern standards, authoritarian tone, in that Hartland appeared to be giving instructions rather than suggestions[2]. However, note the importance of the verbal delivery, and the accent placed upon the words here printed in bold type, all of which carry powerful, more covert suggestions.

Note too Hartland's use of repetition, which establishes a rhythm to the delivery, deepening the trance and further potentiating the suggestions. Finally, note the use of alliteration and assonance, particularly in the phrasing "**stronger and steadier** … your mind **calmer and clearer** … **more composed** … **more placid** … **more tranquil** …".

> *"You have now become* **so** *deeply relaxed …* **so** *deeply asleep … that your mind has become* **so** *sensitive …* **so** *… receptive to what I say … that* **everything** *that I put into your mind … will sink* **so** *deeply into the unconscious part of your mind … and will cause* **so** *deep and lasting an impression there … that* **nothing** *will eradicate it.*
>
> *Consequently … these things that I put into your unconscious mind … will begin to exercise a greater and greater influence over the way you think … over the way you feel … over the way you behave.*
>
> *And … because these things* **will** *remain … firmly embedded in the unconscious part of your mind … after you have left here … when you are no longer with me … they will continue to exercise that same great influence … over your* **thoughts** *… your* **feelings** *… and your* **actions** *…* **just** *as strongly …* **just** *as surely …* **just** *as powerfully … when you are back home … or at work … as when you are with me in this room.*
>
> *You are now so* **very deeply asleep** *… that* **everything** *I tell you is going to happen to you …* **for your own good** *…* **will** *happen exactly as I tell you.*
>
> *And* **every feeling** *… that I tell you that you will experience … you will experience … exactly as I tell you.*
>
> *And these same things will continue to happen to you … every day … and you will continue to experience these same feelings … every day … just as strongly … just as surely … just as powerfully … when you are back home … or at work … as when you are with me in this room.*
>
> *During this deep sleep … you are going to feel physically* **stronger** *and* **fitter** *in every way. You will feel* **more alert** *…* **more wide awake** *… more energetic. You will become* **much less** *easily tired …* **much less** *easily fatigued …* **much less** *easily discouraged …* **much less** *easily depressed.* **Every day** *… you will become so deeply* **interested** *in whatever you're doing … in whatever is going on around you … that your mind will become* **completely distracted away from yourself.**

You will no longer think nearly as much about yourself ... you will no longer dwell at nearly as much upon yourself and your difficulties ... and you will become much less conscious of yourself ... much less preoccupied with yourself ... and with your own feelings.

Every day ... your nerves will become stronger and steadier ... your mind calmer and clearer ... more composed ... more placid ... more tranquil. You will become much less easily worried ... much less easily agitated ... much less easily fearful and apprehensive ... much less easily upset.

You will be able to **think more clearly** *... you will be able to* **concentrate more easily.**

You will be able to give up your whole undivided attention to whatever you are doing ... to the complete exclusion of everything else. Consequently your memory will rapidly improve ... and you will be able to see things in their true perspective ... without magnifying your difficulties ... without ever allowing them to get out of proportion.

Every day ... you will become emotionally much calmer ... much more settled ... much less easily disturbed.

Every day ... *you* **will become ...** *and* **you** *will remain ...* **more and more completely relaxed** *...* **and less tense** *each day ...* **both mentally and physically** *... even when you are no longer with me.*

And **as** *you become ...* **and as** *you remain ...* **more relaxed** *...* **and less tense** *each day ... so you will develop* **much more confidence in yourself** *... more confidence in your ability to* **do** *... not only what you* **have** *... to do each day but more confidence in your ability to do whatever you ought to be able to do ...* **without fear of failure ... without fear of consequences ... without unnecessary anxiety ... without uneasiness.**

Because of this ... every day ... you will feel more and more independent ... more able to 'stick up' for yourself ... to stand upon your own feet ... to hold your own ... no matter how difficult or trying things may be.

Every day ... you will feel a greater feeling of personal well-being ... a greater feeling of personal safety ... and security ... than you have felt for a long, long time.

And because all these things **will** *begin to happen ...* **exactly** *as I tell you they will happen ...* **more and more rapidly ... powerfully ... and completely** *... with every treatment I give you ... you will feel* **much happier ... much more contented ... much more optimistic** *in every way.*

You will consequently become much more able to **rely upon ... to depend upon ...** *yourself ...* **your own efforts ... your own judgement ... your own opinions.** *You will feel much less need ... to have to* **rely upon ... or to depend upon ...** *other people."*

Ego-strengthening (after M. Heap)

Note here the modern, more permissive and less prescriptive approach[4]:

"As you are relaxing and letting go, you may at some time be considering how many things you have learnt to do and how you learnt to do those things – everyday things like reading and writing, walking and talking, for instance ... You have now learnt to do all these things automatically, so now you don't even have to try to do them ...

Now as you're relaxing ... and each time you relax like this, either with me or on your own, you can be learning just from the experience ... how to relax and be calm in everyday situations, not just when you are sitting or lying down, but also when you are up and about and active ... how to feel in control so when you do start to experience any anxious thoughts and feelings, you can control them ... they won't control you.

You are learning all this from the experience of relaxing, in the same way that you have learnt so many things just by experiencing them ... and as you are learning that you can control these anxious thoughts and feelings, so you will find it easier and easier to put aside these thoughts and feelings when they do arise ... just like when someone's trying to bother you and distract you and you ignore them and carry on with what you're doing – they soon go away, and you don't even notice when they have gone.

So any time you are aware of any unnecessary thoughts or feelings of anxiety or self-doubt, you can think to yourself "I can control them. They won't control me!" and you can immediately switch your attention away from yourself and towards whatever you are doing and whatever is happening around you ... and it might surprise you when you realise sometime later that those anxious thoughts and feelings have gone away.

So in this way you can start to feel more confident in your ability to handle any tense or anxious thoughts and feelings and any doubts about yourself ... so, you will feel more confident to face up to things and enter situations which previously you may have avoided ... feeling more calm, more in control and more ready to take on the things that you wish to do ... Do the things you want to do ... Say the things you want to say ... in your own way. You can be learning all this as you are relaxing ... just from the experience of relaxing.

So just continue to relax for a little longer and imagine all these suggestions finding a place deep down in your mind where they can work automatically and effectively whenever you need them in your everyday life."

The use of guided imagery in ego-strengthening

By the use of guided imagery you can direct a patient to take a different view of their situation with a corresponding increase in their self-esteem and sense of control:

[not to be used with a patient with a flying phobia!]

"... I wonder if you've ever been about to travel by plane on a really cloudy day ... and as you look upwards the clouds are low and dark and threatening ... almost as if there's a weight of cloud hanging above your head ... almost like a pressure above you and then there's a smooth

acceleration and take off ... and you climb ... and soon you are in the clouds ... just like a fog ... and then suddenly you are through and above those clouds ... and the sunlight is so bright ... and the sky an intense blue ... and the clouds are below you ... dazzling white ... like snow with occasional dazzling white icebergs ... and you know that they are the same clouds that you saw from below ... which looked so dark and oppressive ... the very same clouds that you are now looking down on.

And I guess that can happen with all sorts of things ... that problems are above you ... dark ... pressing down ... but when you make that flight of imagination ... you can soar through ... and start looking at those same problems from above ... far below you ... and suddenly you are in control of them ... above them ... strong ... more confident and clear headed ... able to make choices and decisions ..."

Five-step approach (H. Stanton)

Stanton[5] describes a five step approach to ego-strengthening within which visual imagery is incorporated. The script here incorporated (G.T.) is given as an example.

1) **Create as much physical relaxation as feasible**.
    "I would like you to become more aware of your breathing ... noting the air passing smoothly into your lungs, and then flowing out ... and imagine as that air flows out, all the tension in your body starts to flow out with it ... feel it draining out ... with each breath ... begin to let go of any discomfort ... let go of any problems, worries ... each time you exhale ... letting go ... feeling more and more relaxed ..."

2) **Introduce the concept of the mind as a pond**, the conscious part above the surface and the unconscious below. Suggest that the patient then imagines a beautiful stone representing, for instance, calmness. As this stone slowly sinks deeper and deeper until it rests at the bottom, the calmness becomes a permanent part of their life. This procedure can be repeated with other stones representing other qualities or suggestions.
    "... Now imagine that your mind is a pond ... with the surface perfectly calm and still ... like a mirror ... with the area above the surface as your conscious thoughts ... and that below as the deeper, unconscious part of your mind ... and as you look close to the side of this pond you become aware of some stones ... and the interesting thing is ... each of theses stones represents some quality that you would find very helpful to you ... it may be that these qualities are written on the stones ... or they may be engraved, so that when you touch the stones you can feel that quality ... or they may even somehow speak to you ... and what is really wonderful ... is that, as you drop a stone into that pond ... and as that stone sinks gently down ... deeper, and deeper ... until it reaches the bottom of the pond ... that quality spreads throughout your mind ... so ... find the stone that represents Calmness ... and drop it into the pond ... be aware of it sinking gently down ... deeper and deeper ... and as it rests gently on the bottom ... feel that Calmness spreading throughout your mind ... gradually becoming a permanent part of your

life ... now take the stone that represents Control ... and as that stone sinks down ... reaching the bottom ... feel that control begin to spread ... and it's so good to look forward to ... being more in control ... over your thoughts ... feelings ... and behaviour ..."

3) Propose that the patient can then dispose of all unwanted feelings, attitudes and behaviour.

"... and near to the pond there is some running water ... maybe a stream ... maybe a river ... and you can go to the side where it is safe ... and imagine ... that you have all your mental 'rubbish' there ... and imagine all that 'rubbish' – it may be in bags or just scattered about ... imagine dumping all of it ... easily throwing, or letting it slide into the water ... to be carried away ... forever ... all your doubts ... fears ... guilt ... no need to examine it, just feel so glad that you are getting rid of it ... feeling such a relief ... to let go of all that weight ... as all your 'rubbish' floats away ... never to return ..."

4) Now suggest that patients imagine that they are removing a barrier that represents everything negative in their lives.

"... so, feeling more in control ... and stronger ... you can be aware of a barrier ... and this barrier is made up of all the things that have prevented you from being how you want to be ... from doing the things you want to do ... feeling how you want to feel ... the negative thoughts, self-imposed limits, all your fears and worries, are making up this barrier ... but now you are ready to smash this barrier ... so you can take a sledgehammer [or a laser, robot – whatever may be appropriate for that patient] *and demolish that barrier ... giving yourself the freedom ... to move on ..."*

5) Lastly, invite the patient to go to their "special place". This concept is widely used in a variety of ways.

"... and as you move on ... I would like you to imagine a door ... and let yourself through that door ... and close it behind you ... leaving the rest of the world behind ... so that you can visit your own 'special place' ... just for you ... a place where you feel so very calm and relaxed ... safe and secure ... so content ... this place may be somewhere that you know well ... or it may be somewhere that you would like to visit ... or it may be somewhere that you simply imagine ... but wherever it is ... this 'special place' is where you can feel totally relaxed ... safe and secure ... where you can imagine yourself doing all the things you want to do ... behaving just as you would want to behave ... allowing your unconscious mind to sort out all the issues that need dealing with ... leaving you to feel relaxed and calm ... at peace ... perhaps forgetting all about things that used to bother you ... because these things seem so much less important to you now ... and when things become less important, the memory of those things fades away ..."

The "pond", "rubbish chute" and "barrier" all rely on the patient using their imagination, generating their own variations and modifications to be truly effective. This is preferable to feeding the patient a standard script that may not consistently fit in with their personally constructed imagery.

14

Ideomotor Signalling

When we are communicating with another person we constantly give involuntary non-verbal signals. We may nod or shake our head without conscious awareness, showing our agreement or disagreement with whatever it is our partner is expressing, and the unconscious smile or frown will often give a very clear message of our emotional response to a situation. In hypnosis ideomotor responses are defined as responses in which internal thoughts and ideas, agreement and disagreement, are translated into such movements[6]. In effect you teach the patient a specific set of responses by which they can communicate without having to speak. Most patients will find this very acceptable, preferring not to speak during hypnosis as the effort of so doing may disturb their pleasant state of relaxation.

An essential characteristic of these responses is that having learnt them the patient will then perceive them as taking place involuntarily, without conscious effort playing a part in the movement. Ideomotor signalling is a valuable adjunct in the majority of hypnotic interventions, allowing communication that deepens rather than breaks the hypnotic flow. Among its benefits are:

- To allow the patient to recognise that they have an element of control over the dental procedure. For many patients this control factor is of fundamental importance in reducing anxiety.
- To clarify uncertain aspects of the patient's history. Conventionally this history will have been gleaned by the use of open questioning. The use of closed questions in the hypnotic state will allow both the patient and yourself greater insight into specific relevant areas.
- To facilitate a hypnotic desensitisation programme or cognitive behavioural therapy. In a number of therapeutic modes the patient may be asked to enter certain imaginary situations, and ideomotor signalling of their progress is of paramount importance for their comfort and safety.

In investigative and psychodynamic therapies the ideomotor response is an indicator of progress and can also be used as a "get out" if the patient finds the experience intolerable.

Advantages of an ideomotor signalling system

It can act in its own right as an induction process. Some patients will, when given the instructions to set up the response (see below), automatically close their eyes and enter a light hypnotic state. If this occurs no further induction suggestions may be necessary.

The lethargy of the hypnotic state will often make it difficult for the patient to verbalise an answer to a question and in trying to do so the state will almost inevitably be lightened. By eliminating the effort of thought and speech the depth of hypnosis can be maintained and deepened.

The perception of involuntariness is important as it demonstrates that something different and special is happening in hypnosis – increasing its mystique. This will facilitate therapy and also act as a deepening device.

The closed question format necessitated by ideomotor signalling allows you to target questions in order to produce specific and concise answers.

The suggestions given can be structured to allow the patient to give an honest response without having consciously to *try* to think of an acceptable answer, thus increasing the likelihood of a genuinely felt response.

Although a skilled therapist may be able to use other responses, such as changes in breathing rates, muscle tension and facial colour and/or facial expression as indications of patients' responses to questioning, a finger signal is easier to note.

It gives the patient a perception of control and involvement in their therapy, and indeed the security of being able to "stop the action" in the dental setting in the event of their feeling uncomfortable.

Setting up and using an ideomotor signalling response

Preparing the patient

Before inducing hypnosis it is important that the patient is told what to expect. Note that these scripts are simply a guide. Your delivery will depend upon the nature of the patient, and as you work you should gradually move into your "hypnotic" voice. In fact, for many patients this script, when delivered in a slow rhythmic style, will act as an induction process.

Note also that the whole process which follows takes only a little more time than it does simply to read it.

Introducing the ideomotor response

"Have you noticed that often when you're talking to someone they nod or shake their head at what your saying, without even realising that they're doing it? We all smile or frown quite unconsciously when we like or dislike something. When people talk about making a phone call they often raise their hand quite unconsciously as if they're holding a phone. So in everyday life we communicate using our bodies as well as words; we use hand gestures and head movements unconsciously ... without thinking.

Soon you are going to be enjoying really deep relaxation in hypnosis [pre-hypnotic suggestion], *and although you will be able to speak if you want to, you'll probably be happier to just stay deeply relaxed without even making the effort. So what we're going to do is set up a system by which you can signal 'yes' or 'no' to me by using your fingers, without even having to think about it. Is that OK with you? ... Good. Let's make a start."*

Induction

Use a rapid induction procedure such as a simple eye roll if necessary. There is rarely any need at this stage to go through any deepening procedure.

Positioning the hand

In the dental setting the left hand is preferable to the right for the purpose of signalling. This is because from the normal seated position of the patient that hand is in your direct sight-line, and at the same time you are allowed clear vision of the patient's face and body so that any other non-verbal cues such as grimacing or altered breathing pattern are easily observable.

The patient's hand and arm should first be positioned on the armrest of the chair; by slightly flexing the elbow, the hand can be raised and maintained a few inches above the armrest. This will make any finger movement even more noticeable.

The signalling system

"Now what we're going to do is to allow your fingers on that left hand ... I'm just touching that hand now ... [gently touch the hand].. *to communicate with me just like nodding or shaking your head ... and you won't need to even think about it because you'll find it will just happen automatically. Let's start by just allowing yourself to think of the word 'yes' ... keep saying to yourself 'yes, yes, yes' ... and as you do so I wonder which finger your unconscious mind will choose to represent 'yes'. When it has done so, you'll find that one of your*

fingers, or perhaps your thumb, will lift up, all by itself, to let me know which one has been chosen. I wonder which one it's going to be ..."

[After a variable length of time, often just a few seconds, one of the patient's fingers will start to flicker.]

"... and I can see that your unconscious mind has chosen that finger as your 'yes' finger ... that's brilliant ... just let it rise on its own so that we both know that that is your 'yes' finger ...[touch the finger gently at this stage] ... so that if at any time here I ask you a question and your unconscious mind ... that special part at the back of your mind ... wants to answer 'yes' ... that 'yes' finger will flicker and rise just as it has done just now.

And now let that finger just drop back down to where it was before, and as it does so let yourself become even more deeply relaxed" [deepening procedure].

Then go through the same routine for selection of the "no" finger. Note again that the finger-raising signifying an ideomotor response will be hesitant and flickery. A firmly raised finger is more likely to indicate conscious control by the patient.

If there is no apparent response you may suggest that a change in feeling may be experienced in one of the fingers, rather than movement, and that it is OK to help by moving that finger slightly. This generally starts the process and ideomotor responses will supervene.

It is important once again to identify the respective fingers to the patient, and to make a note for yourself in order to avoid confusion.

Reinforcing and testing the response

"... you've done really well, so allow yourself to relax even more deeply and we'll just look again at the way your unconscious mind has chosen to indicate 'yes' and 'no'... it seems to have chosen this finger [touch] *for 'yes' and this finger* [touch] *for 'no' ... let's just see ... Is your name* [patient's name]? *[the patient's 'yes' finger rises] ... that's great ... and now let that finger just drop back down to where it was before, and as it does so let yourself become even more deeply relaxed ... and another question... Do you live in* [wrong city]? *[the patient's 'no' finger rises] ... that's great ... and now let that finger just drop back down to where it was before, and as it does so let yourself become even more deeply relaxed ... so now we can just let your unconscious mind take over and you can just let yourself become so deeply relaxed ..."*

Further notes

As a general principle, each time the patient has answered a question by ideomotor response it should become a habit to thank them and to suggest that as the finger drops down to its natural position they will become even more deeply relaxed (see section on deepening).

- Your questioning style must be "closed" and absolutely specific. Open questions such as "Do you want me to continue or shall I pause?", or "How are you doing?", or "What's the trouble?", or "Don't you want me to go on?" preclude an ideomotor response, and can cause great confusion and an abundance of conscious effort as the patient struggles to an express an answer non-verbally.

  The simple closed questions "Are you comfortable?", "Is it OK for me to continue?", "Do you want me to stop?", are clear and unambiguous and require a simple "yes" or "no" response.

- Make sure that the patient's hand is positioned in a good sight line when you are in your natural working position.

- Do not rely merely on the ideomotor response, but maintain your awareness of all the other involuntary and unconscious signals the patient may be exhibiting.

- When inducing glove analgesia (see Chapter 25) be certain that the hand used for the ideomotor response is not the hand in which you are inducing analgesia.

- The patient's responses must always immediately be totally respected and accepted. Any failure so to do will break down trust, and probably result in the patient becoming more anxious and less trusting of you and of hypnosis as an adjunct to treatment.

Remember that an ideomotor response is not infallible and cannot be used as a "lie detector"; the patient does in fact have an element of conscious control of the movement.

15

Post-hypnotic Suggestions

Post-hypnotic suggestions are suggestions given in hypnosis in order to produce a response at some time after the patient has been alerted. Generally these suggestions may be simple ideas that link a specific cue with a specific outcome. The cue might be based upon an action, a thought, words or an event, the suggestion being that this specific cue will trigger the desired response:

> *"... from now on as soon as you sit in the dental chair you will become as deeply relaxed as you are now ..."*

or

> *"..in future if you feel anxious you will say to yourself 'calm' as you breathe out, and the anxiety will melt away.."*

Post-hypnotic suggestions are a fundamental element in clinical hypnosis, empowering the patient to change his responses and behaviour wherever and whenever it is necessary. For example, a person feeling anxious about a dental appointment would employ suitable post-hypnotic suggestion to reduce that anxiety without the need for further hypnosis at that time. You will give the suggestion to the relaxed patient in hypnosis that if at any future time he feels the anxiety, by taking slow deep breaths he can restore those same feelings of calm, relaxation and control.

Post-hypnotic suggestions can often be effective with a single delivery, but repetition, both in that session and in subsequent sessions of auto-hypnosis or hetero-hypnosis, will reinforce the effect. It is important then that the patient practises the technique, in effect developing a conditioned response to the suggested cue.

As with any form of suggestion, the effectiveness of post-hypnotic suggestions will vary. The outcome will depend largely upon the patient's hypnotic talent, but other factors involved will be their motivation, the relevance of any cues and whether the suggestions are specific and make sense to that patient at that time.

Although popular culture – for instance in the novel *Trilby* – depicts post-hypnotic suggestions being used by unscrupulous hypnotists to persuade their subject to carry out criminal and immoral acts, this is far from the case. In fact post-hypnotic suggestions are analogous to the normal suggestions given in hypnosis, in that the patient may ignore or override them unless the suggestions encompass their therapeutic needs at that time.

Time and situation specificity

It is fundamental that any post-hypnotic suggestions are time and situation specific. This is best achieved by routinely using a formula that links occasion, cue and outcome. For example:
- *occasion:* "... if you feel that anxious feeling in your stomach ..."
- *cue:* "... you will count three gentle outgoing breaths ..."
- *outcome:* "... and the feelings will just melt away."

It is recognised that post-hypnotic suggestions given towards the end of a session are taken up more readily than those given at the beginning of a session, and can often be part of the alerting procedure.

> *"... seven ... quite soon I will be asking you to open your eyes ...*
>
> *... eight ... knowing that at any time in future ... if you feel that anxious feeling in your stomach ... you will simply count three gentle outgoing breaths ... and the feelings will just melt away ...*
>
> *... nine ... feeling more and more alert ... relaxed yet alert ... increasingly back in touch with where you are here at the dental practice with me ... and ten ... eyes open ... wide awake ... alert ... ready to get on with your day."*

Post-hypnotic suggestion as an induction method

Post-hypnotic suggestions can be used extremely effectively in facilitating subsequent hypnotic induction.

> *"Any time in the future you wish to experience this comfortable, pleasant state of relaxation, all you need to do is take ten deep, slow breaths, and by the time you reach the tenth breath, you will be pleased to find that your eyelids have closed, and you are drifting into this wonderful state of relaxed, focused awareness."*

Or:

> *"When you next come here for treatment you will notice yourself becoming more relaxed ... and as soon as you are seated ... and the chair is adjusted ... you can allow your eyes to close and enjoy these same feelings of relaxation, comfort and being in control."*

In anxiety management

> *"... and if at any time in the future you feel those anxious feelings in your stomach and your chest ... or in your mind ... you'll imagine that colour of anxiety that you told me about ... and as you breathe out you'll imagine gently blowing away that colour ... that anxiety ... and your body and mind will start to feel calm and comfortable again ..."*

To manage denture intolerance

"... in future ... you'll find that when you are about to put your upper denture into your mouth ... you'll have a flashback memory of how relaxed and comfortable you are now ... and the denture will feel really good in your mouth ... and you'll feel so good knowing you look so much better ..."

In pain management

Patients may sometimes describe pain as "coming in waves", and often their response to the wave of pain is to tense up, frequently making the pain worse. The following technique can be learned:

"... just imagine how water flows through a clear pipe ... and imagine that if that pain were to come again it could flow right through you and flow away ... if you take a really deep breath ... and hold it ... and as the pain comes ... let your breath out ... just flowing away ... just as the pain flows away with your breath ... flows right away ..."

A further important use of post-hypnotic suggestions is in pain management by self-analgesia (see Chapter 25). Here the patient is taught in hypnosis to transfer analgesia from a finger to a tooth, following which at a later appointment the suggestion might be:

"... I'm going to be working on that tooth at the front of your mouth ... [touching the tooth with a probe] ... so what I'd like you to do now is to rub that tooth and the area around it ... and when you know it is numb please drop your hand down ... and go into even deeper relaxation while I do the work ..."

16

Anchoring

An "anchor" is a sensory input, real or imaginary, that is inevitably linked to an emotion. The sensory input may be by sound, sight, taste, smell or touch, and memory of just one part of the input can spontaneously bring back the entire image including the emotion, which may be positive or negative.

The term "anchoring" was popularised in the context of NLP by Bandler and Grinder[7] to describe the phenomenon of paired association, whereby an external stimulus produces an internal feeling as a *conditioned response*. Much of our behaviour is governed by conditioned responses, as is our response to many of the stimuli with which we come into contact.

For example, how many couples go gooey-eyed (or not!) when they hear "our tune"? The powerful ability of a smell to link us by reflex to a past experience has been widely used by department stores and supermarkets, which will place perfume displays or freshly baked bread strategically to set up an appropriate emotional response as customers enter the store.

Anchoring also has a negative side, and this can be a very important factor in maintaining habits and phobias. The words we use and even the smell of a surgery can act as negative anchors. To a dental phobic the mention of a root canal or even the word "dentist", or the mere hint of the smell of disinfectant, can produce an overwhelming response of autonomic arousal leading, again by conditioned response, to a panic attack. A patient may even develop a negative anchor based upon the smell of a dental surgeon's aftershave. Many people being treated with chemotherapy develop a pre-treatment anticipatory nausea, and this may persist even after all treatment if they happen to walk by the oncology hospital.

But in a positive sense anchoring is a way in which we can teach the patient a conditioned response as a safe anchor for their emotions when they are drifting negatively into anxiety and fear in the dental surgery. For treatment to be successful the patient's negative anchors are therapeutically dismantled and replaced with more helpful ones, and hypnosis is an ideal vehicle for carrying this out.

The process

Setting up a positive anchor

In hypnosis invite the patient to access a past experience when pleasant, confident, positive feelings were present, and ask them to affirm that this is happening by nodding their head or by an agreed ideomotor signal. Through hypnotic suggestion intensify those feelings, until the patient signals that they are imagining the event as vividly as possible.

At this point invite the patient to set up a physical link, the *anchoring stimulus*, with these feelings. This link may take the form of you placing a hand on the patient's shoulder, or an action taken by the patient such as a clenching their fist. Suggestions are then made to link together the physical action with the emotional state being experienced at that time.

By the use of repetition the patient quickly develops a *reflex* loop linking the physical action with the appropriate emotion. You can then encourage the patient in hypnosis to experience the original negative stimulus and to interrupt it by the newly acquired anchor. The patient is then encouraged to practice the technique repeatedly, and instruction in self-hypnosis can be used as a *reinforcer*.

Summary of technique for anchoring
- Induce and deepen trance.
- Ask the patient to access a memory of some event where the desired qualities such as calm, confidence and control were present. Obtain a response from the patient to confirm this.
- Suggest that the patient then recreates that memory as vividly as possible, using all their senses. Get confirmation of this.
- Establish the anchor by pressing the patient's shoulder or by asking them to clench their fist.
- Suggest that each time they experience this signal, they will *automatically* bring back those feelings.
- Repeat this process several times with different memories if possible.
- If the patient is to use self-hypnosis, instruct them to practice this repeatedly.
- Introduce ego-strengthening and post-hypnotic instruction for self-hypnosis.
- Alert.

Notes

The image must be appropriate for that person and for their needs at that particular time (not everyone likes beaches or walking through gardens).

You might suggest "... somewhere maybe you have visited, or where you would like to be, or where you feel content and comfortable ... might be indoors or outdoors ... might be alone or with someone else ... might even be fantasy ...".

Use your skills to facilitate the quality of the scene, but there is no need for you to know what it is, unless the patient volunteers this or asks for your help in accessing an image. Remember too that the patient's image may be very personal and intimate ... do not get involved.

Note that the aim is to create a conditioned response as a result of which firing the anchor in the patient's waking state will bring back the resourceful feelings, but not necessarily the fantasised scenes and *not* the trance.

Examples of anchoring

Hand on shoulder
Because of the nature of dentistry and the relative position of patient and dentist, a hand on the patient's shoulder is a natural form of reassurance whether or not you are using hypnosis. Nevertheless, there are some patients for whom this form of physical contact is not comfortable, and you should always use your discretion when considering this approach. Having ascertained that it is appropriate, continue as follows.

Induce hypnosis and invite the patient to go to their "safe place" in imagery, and to access and intensify all the feelings of calm, comfort, control, and confidence. Ask them to affirm by an agreed ideomotor signal the moment that they reach a peak in the desired feelings, and watch carefully. At the instant that they signal place your hand on their shoulder with a firm pressure and gently squeeze for about 5 seconds, then remove your hand. Repeat this exercise four or five times.

Thereafter, at future appointments use the anchor quite naturally in order to trigger those feelings in the patient, whether or not you are using hypnosis.

"Power at your fingertips"
The following example requires that you touch the patient's wrist. Remember that whenever hypnosis involves touching the patient it is necessary to obtain their permission before starting treatment.

When the patient is in hypnosis and suitably relaxed you can intensify that feeling:

> *"When I lift your hand by the wrist, feel how heavy and relaxed your arm and hand are becoming ... and as I let it drop down onto your leg I wonder how much more relaxed it will become, each time your arm drops it feels more and more loose and relaxed, as you feel more and more calm, and comfortable."*
>
> [Drop and lift up the patient's arm a few times, making suggestions to reinforce the desired feelings, until you feel that they are sufficiently relaxed. Now proceed to create the anchor.]
>
> *"As you continue to feel so relaxed, comfortable and calm ... I'd like you to rub a finger and thumb of one hand together ... and you may be surprised to discover that from now on, every time that you rub those fingers together ... you will start to feel calm, comfortable and relaxed, just as you are now ... whenever you need to be."*

These anchors can often be established the first time they are set up, although repeating the procedure will reinforce their effect.

The patient should keep rubbing for 20 to 30 seconds before being allowed to rest, and they are reminded that they can access those feelings at any time in the future. Now ask the patient to repeat the process as you reinforce the suggestions for calm, control and relaxation. As a further endorsement you might give a post-hypnotic suggestion for regular practice of the procedure.

Clenched fist technique (after Calvert Stein)

With this technique[8], following induction, deepening and accessing appropriate feelings:

1) Ask the patient to clench the fist of their dominant hand and suggest that they:

   "... imagine holding all those good images and feelings in that hand ... aware that you now have a grip on your feelings ... and you know that those feelings are ready at hand ... at any time."

2) Ask the patient then to release that fist and impress on them that they can access those feelings any time that they clench that fist. Get them to rehearse this exercise several times.

3) As a further endorsement you might give a post-hypnotic suggestion for regular practice of the procedure.

This procedure can be extended. Invite the patient to return in their mind to the situation that is at the centre of their fear:

> *"... and experience that situation as vividly as you feel you can at this time ... become immersed in it ... feel those feelings ... and now ... make a fist with your non-dominant hand ... and imagine all the tension and other bad feelings flowing down into that fist ... and as those feelings flow down ... the fist gets tighter and tighter ... and even though the rest of your body remains deeply comfortable and relaxed ... and you continue to breathe steadily ... that fist gets tighter and tighter as it grasps all those bad feelings ..."*
>
> *"now ... as you unclench that fist and let it relax ... imagine letting go of all that tension ... and begin to feel the good, positive feelings and all their resources and strengths coming in that situation as you clench your dominant hand into a fist. Keep that hand clenched until the other hand is fully open and relaxed, and now start to feel so confident and in control."*

Ask the patient to repeat the exercise, at the same time giving post-hypnotic suggestions that they rehearse it imagining themselves using the technique successfully and experiencing themselves coping really well in any future situations.

The use of sound

Anchors can involve any of the senses. For instance, it is possible to use the sound of the dental drill as a positive anchor. As before, the first stage is to ensure that the patient is as relaxed as possible before proceeding;

> "... *from now on, whenever you hear this sound* ... [activate the drill] ... *you will find yourself becoming just as calm and relaxed as you are today* ... *and this sound may remind you of a piece of music you really enjoy* ... *or the sound of the plane taking you on holiday* ...
> [tailor ideas appropriate to the patient's fantasy] ... *helping you to remain calm, in control, relaxed* ... *every time you hear this sound.*"

Operate the drill for about 10 seconds, and then after a short rest repeat this. After hypnosis, you can test the effect of the procedure by operating the drill and noting the patient's reaction.

17

Self-hypnosis

Self hypnosis, also referred to as *auto-hypnosis*, is a means by which a patient is able to use hypnosis at a time of their own choosing in order to take charge of their own therapy and to reinforce the various suggestions and post-hypnotic suggestions that you have made. It can be regarded as a natural extension of the *hetero-hypnosis* that you carry out in your surgery.

Through self-hypnosis the dental patient establishes autonomy and independence, so that by the inclusion of appropriate ego-strengthening suggestions they will develop the self-confidence to visit either yourself or any other dentist for future treatment.

For some the idea of entering hypnosis might be in itself quite intimidating, and many people are also self-conscious about their ability to deal with the process. You should emphasise to the patient that entering and using hypnosis is an acquired skill, and that your own role may be seen as that of a teacher or guide. As with any skill practice will inevitably produce improvement, and so by using self-hypnosis the patient can gain confidence and expertise, consequently finding that when they return their improved skills and confidence can greatly facilitate the process of dental treatment.

The majority of patients will not initially achieve the same depth when in self-hypnosis as when experiencing hypnosis with you, as they cannot relinquish conscious control to the same extent as when with a trusted ally. In part this is due to the fact that the patient is having to play the two roles of patient and therapist simultaneously. In other words he must be active and passive at the same time, going through the mental working in hypnosis while at the same time observing himself as though from the outside. Nevertheless, with practice the increase in confidence allows the conscious observing role to diminish and the hypnosis to become deeper.

There will occasionally be patients who find it difficult to concentrate and to dissociate themselves sufficiently to enter self-hypnosis. In these cases the use of individualised tape-recordings or CDs of induction and therapy can be of immense value, and this will be looked at in more detail elsewhere in this chapter.

Some uses of self hypnosis

Self-hypnosis can be used to supplement and enhance any suggestions that you have made within a patient's treatment. The following are some common examples.

To reduce anxiety and stress

Dr Johannes Schultz (see page 10) noted that patients who simply carried out verbal self-hypnosis instructions experienced a state of heaviness, well-being and warmth, and that physical concerns such as headaches and fatigue would often disappear[9]. By extension, for many people the use of a self-hypnosis relaxation routine can in a very short space of time produce these same improvements in general well-being, decreased anxiety and lessening of symptoms.

To reinforce therapy

Self-hypnosis can replicate the work that you and the patient have done together in any hypnosis sessions. For example the patient can maintain their motivation to stop smoking, or to reinforce any anchors established.

To increase self-control

Self-hypnosis can give people a greater sense of control over their thoughts, feelings and behaviour. This can be valuable in the development of their autonomy, and also when attempting to eradicate habits such as bruxism.

In developing and using imagery

Any imagery that has been used in therapy can be repeated, enhanced and developed. For example, the patient might rehearse the fantasy of going to the dentist and experiencing any treatment comfortably and successfully. Future pacing is almost inevitably linked to self-hypnosis.

In pain control

Any techniques found to be successful in controlling pain and discomfort can be practised in self hypnosis. As well as the obvious comfort that the patient will achieve, self-hypnosis will allow the patient a sense of autonomy and lessened dependency upon chemical pain control.

Setting up self-hypnosis

Generally it is helpful to instruct the patient in self-hypnosis early on in their treatment, sometimes even at their first visit. It is always important first to ensure that the patient is sufficiently comfortable with hypnosis, and that the procedures chosen to be used to enter self-hypnosis are the most effective for that person as an individual.

Teaching self-hypnosis in the form of post-hypnotic suggestions is possibly the simplest way, and it is sensible to avoid any induction methods that employ more extravagant physical actions such as hand or arm levitation as this would usually inhibit the patient from using self-hypnosis at times of acute need when in a public place.

Most patients will not require an elaborate ritual for their self-hypnosis induction – in fact the simpler the process the better – but setting up a specific routine makes the whole regime much easier, and by repetition reinforces the habit. When the patient has once become more confident, comfortable and at ease with the process, a simple trigger word such as "calm" or an action such as a clenched fist can be introduced, and this may be used as an anchor for a specific therapeutic purpose, for instance in aborting a panic attack.

It is sensible to explain to the patient in their normal wakened state that you are going to teach them self-hypnosis, and then to teach the specific techniques while the patient is in hypnosis, as in this way the instructions will be readily absorbed. After the self-hypnosis has been taught, the patient should be allowed to demonstrate that they can successfully enter hypnosis on their own, while you observe and encourage them.

Sometimes the patient may report unexpected effects that they have experienced when using hypnosis. These may include physical sensations such as tingling or heaviness, or diverse images or feelings. You might use any such descriptions to validate the quality of their experience, and then suggest that the patient uses these sensations in order to deepen the hypnotic state.

General points regarding self-hypnosis

Some people seem to be able to read, daydream or catnap wherever they are. For such people self-hypnosis will probably be easy to attain no matter how distracting their surroundings. However, the majority will find it necessary, especially for their early attempts, to practise self-hypnosis with a minimum of distraction. So the recommendation would be to find somewhere relatively quiet and private, where there is as little noise from outside as possible and the chances of being disturbed are reduced.

In order to enter and successfully use self-hypnosis it is important to feel comfortable, safe and secure whether one is seated or lying down, though in most situations a seat is much more accessible than a bed or a couch. People using a bed may find that they drift off to sleep, although – particularly when symptoms have included insomnia – this may be a highly desirable response.

If the patient is seated, their head should be well supported in order that their neck and shoulder muscles remain comfortable during relaxation. Their feet would normally be flat on the floor to support the weight of the legs, but the main consideration is that the person is as comfortable as possible.

It should be noted that there will be occasions where "instant" self-hypnosis techniques are used in managing acute traumatic circumstances, and patients should be encouraged to practise such techniques in a normal standing position. Techniques will be described later in this section and can also be found within the section on "anchoring".

In order to gain the benefits of self-hypnosis, regular practice is essential. As with all behaviour, constant use will make it habitual, allowing the patient to enter hypnosis more easily and more quickly so that the benefits of using self-hypnosis will increase.

A concern sometimes expressed is "What if I can't come out of hypnosis?" A useful suggestion to reassure the patient might be: "Trust your unconscious mind to alert you when the time you have allotted to self-hypnosis has elapsed. It will not allow you to remain in trance any longer than is beneficial for you."

Patients may ask when is the best time for them to use self-hypnosis. Obviously for the anxious dental patient, a time shortly before their appointment will be extremely helpful. Rossi describes the *ultradian* rhythms, the natural daily resting phases of the biological cycle, as the "windows of opportunity" for hypnotic intervention[10]. This suggests that certain times during the day are better for practice of self-hypnosis, and also defines the optimum time that such sessions should last as being 20 and 30 minutes. Within this concept optimal times of the day for using self-hypnosis would seem to be after the midday meal, or late in the afternoon, but ultimately it will depend on the patient's lifestyle and timetable. It is usually not a good idea to practise self-hypnosis at bedtime unless sleep is the desired result.

Sometimes people may say that they feel disappointed with their self-hypnosis, claiming that they do not "go as deep as when you do it with me". It is helpful to reassure them by advising them that each time they experience hypnosis it may be to a different depth, and to "trust your unconscious mind to know exactly the right level of trance for you at that particular time".

It is also helpful to explain that it is natural for the mind sometimes to wander, and that this is an indication that the relaxation is becoming a more natural behaviour. By encouraging the patient you are ensuring that they are more likely to persevere.

Self-hypnosis techniques

In general you can teach a patient self-hypnosis as a natural sequel to a normal session of hypnosis in the dental surgery.

> *"Now I'm going to show you how you can take yourself off into this comfortable state just as it is now ... you will find it really helpful to practise this technique until it becomes quite natural and easy to you ... and then you'll be able to use it whenever you like in order to deal with your problem ...*
>
> *What I'd like you to do is to make time for yourself and organise things so that you won't be disturbed ... take the phone off the hook and let everyone know that this is your time. Whether you are sitting down or lying down, get yourself really comfortable, and be prepared just to let go ...*
>
> *You'll know that if anything should happen while you are using self-hypnosis that needs your attention, you'll automatically and instantly be alert and able to respond as necessary ...*

> *in the normal course of events you'll remain aware at the back of your mind of sounds and other things going on around you ... but you'll find that they fade into the background and ... you can simply return in your mind to wherever you were when the disturbance happened ...*
>
> *You'll be aware that each time you use self-hypnosis you will find it easier ... the relaxation will come more quickly, more easily ... and more and more deeply ... and the effects will become stronger and stronger ... and have a beneficial effect over the way you think ... and over the way you feel ... and over the way you behave ...* [here, bring in specific symptom relief where appropriate]
>
> *In a few moments I am going to help you to return to full alertness, and when you do come back to full alertness you'll realise how relaxed you can now become ... you can be really pleased with the way that you've learned how to relax so well ... and know that you can learn how to return to this deep relaxation even when you are on your own ... so now I'd like you to come back to full alertness ... and you can do this by counting slowly to yourself from five down to one, at each stage growing more and more alert ... until at 'one' you will be wide awake ... knowing that you can take yourself back into this deep state of relaxation at any appropriate time simply by using this same method ..."*

The patient should be given these instructions while they are in hypnosis, and encouraged to associate the feelings and images with those experienced during that session. In fact the patient is invited to replicate the induction and process carried out with you, and to try out self-hypnosis immediately after the session while you observe, comment and encourage them.

The imagery suggested below is fairly non-specific, and it should be noted that often you will introduce much more specific suggestions related to the concerns of the patient during the "teaching" session.

Patients should be encouraged to use all their senses, to see, hear, feel, even taste and smell if appropriate, to create as vivid an image as possible.

Some further techniques for self-hypnosis

Counting

> *"So, when you feel ready to go into self-hypnosis, gently close your eyes and let yourself relax ... just as you do when you're here with me ... take a breath, hold it for a few seconds, and then let it out gently ... counting in your mind as you do so one ... two ... three ... and as you do so just allow yourself to relax more and more ... then again, a gentle breath in ... hold it ... and out ... four ... five ... six ... this time going even deeper into the relaxation ... and then once more ... hold your breath for a few seconds and as you breathe out count seven ... eight ... nine ... ten ... and then you can forget about the counting ... and find yourself enjoying*

> *that wonderful feeling of deep relaxation ... and maybe you can let your mind drift into the images that you've found earlier on in this session ... or maybe new happy, safe and secure images ... or maybe just enjoy that beautiful calm, relaxed state ... with your mind drifting wherever it may float off to ... and then ... after a few minutes ... you'll find that you will gently return to being fully alert with your eyes open ... hanging onto all those good, calm feelings ... and all the time you'll know that if anything crops up that needs your attention, you'll automatically and instantly be alert and able to deal with it ... or if you wish to come out of this self-hypnosis at any time ... simply count in your mind ... five ... four ... three ... two ... one and you will open your eyes feeling alert and calm ..."*

Three step eye closure (after David Spiegel)

This is a rapid, reliable technique that avoids the potential pitfalls of challenge. Provided that the patient is willing to go along with what you ask them to do, there is little that can go wrong. The script outlined below can be delivered in a normal conversational style, and the time taken between eye closure and final suggestion is less than half a minute.

> *"... now I'm going to be asking you to take three steps so that you can enter this secure, comfortable state whenever it seems appropriate. It's quite simple, so let's make a start ... for the first stage you will be doing just one thing ... the second two things ... and the third just three things ...*
>
> *... so now ... first just one thing ... roll your eyes upwards ... just as though you're trying to look out of the top of your head ... and second ... two things ... gently close your eyelids over your up-turned eyes ... and take a breath and hold it ... and third, three things ... let that breath out, let your eyes drop to their normal position behind your closed eyelids ... and just let everything go ... and feel yourself sinking down into the chair as you relax more and more deeply ... and find yourself enjoying that wonderful feeling of deep relaxation ..."*
>
> [continue as above]

Eye fixation

> *"... so now please focus your eyes on a point on the wall or the ceiling ... and concentrate on that as closely as possible ... just allow any thoughts that arise to just pass on by, or float away so that you can return to focusing on that spot ... and soon you'll find that your eyelids will flicker and close ... just as they did here today ... and as that happens let yourself just sink down into the chair ... and relax..."*

Clock-face (after Milton Erickson)

> *"... gaze at that wall clock ... and there is movement in the second hand that you can follow with your eyes ... allow your attention to become absorbed in this movement ... notice now your own experience of tension in your body as you focus on the moving second hand ... you can imagine how the gears in the clock are meshing and turning, imagine how the electrical current might be flowing just as energy is flowing in your own body at the same time ... wind yourself up into the focusing experience, and if you find yourself distracted by other thoughts, welcome those thoughts as you remain visually focused on the clock ... you may notice that your heart is beating rapidly, you may even be able to discover a rhythm in the heart beat that is similar or close to the second hand movement ... see if you can find a rhythm and absorb yourself in it."*

Imagery

> *"... and I wonder if you can let yourself go back to a time when you felt calm, relaxed ... absorbed ... confident ... and as you relax you become so deeply involved in that experience that you gently become less aware ... and even unaware of the feelings you had just a little while ago ..."*

Physical changes

In hypnosis you can suggest that the patient experiences an alteration in physical sensation in their hand and arm. This could take the form of heaviness or lightness, warmth or coolness, or a tingling sensation. Encourage the patient then to incorporate this change in sensation into their self-hypnosis session. For example:

> *"As your hand rests comfortably in your lap, you may feel a tingling ... it may be a cool tingling like touching a bottle of chilled white wine, or it may be a warm tingling like holding your hand safely in front of a comforting open fire ... and as you feel that you can allow yourself to go into a deep hypnotic relaxation ..."*

The use of music

Many people can become deeply absorbed in music, and if suitable types of music for that particular patient can be found it can be a great help with self-hypnosis. Although the chosen music will generally be gentle and slow in tempo this is not universally so, and it is most important that the patient chooses something that they like and that they feel is appropriate.

The music can be used as a cue to begin hypnosis, and as it progresses the patient can become so immersed in it that they feel as one with the music, concomitantly becoming dissociated from their surroundings.

Self-hypnosis in acute situations

Often the patient may be relying on self-hypnosis to deal with crises. For example the needle-phobic patient will want to be able to enter hypnosis briefly in order to cope with an injection; a person prone to panic attacks will require a strategy that empowers them to cope in situations when the first sign of impending panic – for instance a lurch of the stomach – arises.

In these situations it is important that the technique works immediately, and also that it is discrete enough to be unnoticed by other people in the vicinity. It is also obviously vital that the patient can carry out the manoeuvre without eye closure, for instance while driving their car!

A simple technique

You can give the patient instruction in abbreviating and simplifying their normal induction procedure together with the option of incorporating eye closure if and when appropriate. This technique can also be combined with a simple anchor as described in Chapter 16.

> *"... if at any time you feel the beginnings of that feeling you told me about, here's what to do ... simply hold your breath for a few seconds ... at the same time bring your special calming word into your mind ... and as you let the breath out feel your body just ease and relax in those few seconds ... as the tension just leaves your body ... and your thoughts and feelings are so much more comfortable ..."*

Anchors

Anchors such as a calming word or the "clenched fist" or "power at your fingertips" are invaluable in helping the patient to deal with acute crises, and are described in Chapter 16.

Safeguards

It is important that patients are given suggestions of reassurance concerning possible interruptions to their self-hypnosis sessions. They may be worried about the possibility of remaining in trance even if an emergency should arise, and thus of being placed in danger. You should advise the patient in hypnosis, while giving their self-hypnosis instruction, that if anything arises that requires their immediate attention they will automatically and instantly be alert and able to respond as necessary.

Whether or not to respond to other distractions can be left to the patient's discretion, and they should be reassured that if they feel it more sensible for them to answer the door bell or the telephone they will do so and then return to hypnosis and be able to continue from where they were when the interruption arose.

Dealing with distraction

Patients may also express concerns about the potential disturbances from the world outside such as passing traffic, police sirens or noisy neighbours. They can be reassured in hypnosis that they will of course hear extraneous noises, but they will find that they are so comfortable and secure that these noises will fade into the background and just be a reminder of their own sense of detachment and comfort.

Alternatively it may be appropriate to suggest incorporating any disturbance into the hypnotic fantasy. For example:

"as you are aware of the sound of a vehicle approaching you can imagine packing up all your tension and worry into a bundle ... and as the sound is closest to you ... throw the bundle into the vehicle to be whisked far away ... and feel that great relief as your tension is carried away ..."

If the patient feels they may be distracted by other sounds, you can suggest that they say to themselves, as appropriate:

"The sound of people talking and enjoying themselves, getting on with their lives, reminds me that I can take time for the important things in my life, such as this self-hypnosis."

"The ticking of the clock reminds me of my heartbeat, strong and steady as I relax and unwind."

Distractions may also be generated internally. It is very difficult, for example, to ignore pain, and so the patient can be taught in hypnosis actually to focus on the pain and begin to use any of the various taught strategies to deal with pain and at the same time to deepen their hypnosis (see Chapter 25).

If the patient finds it hard to stop worrying or doubting, you can suggest that they imagine that they are breathing these fears, worries and doubts away with each exhalation:

"... I wonder if each time you breathe out it can be as though you are gently blowing away those feelings ... maybe you can even see them as having colours ... like a coloured cloud of fear being breathed out and floating away ..."

Use of a recorded CD

Many people adapt easily to a self-hypnosis routine enhanced by a recorded CD or tape. When making a relaxation CD for a patient, appropriate background music can be used to add a natural rhythm to the experience. As well as explaining verbally in advance how to use the CD, an explanatory leaflet may be helpful. (For an example see the Appendix.)

18

The Management of Bleeding

Although the literature is not consistent, there are many studies that show that hypnosis can be used to control bleeding following surgical procedures[11], [12]. In this respect you may recall James Esdaile's observation (see Chapter 1) that the low incidence of surgical shock following his operations was possibly due to the elimination of the stress, pain and accompanying emotional and physiological arousal that the fully conscious patient would have experienced. The concomitant reduction in heart rate and blood pressure doubtless contributed to the dramatic decrease in blood loss experienced.

When suggesting decreased blood flow to an area it is important to let the patient ensure that there is sufficient bleeding to allow the socket to be full so that there will be sufficient tissue present for healing, and the risk of infection is reduced.

Methods

Direct suggestion

Simple direct suggestions to limit the amount of bleeding following treatment may be all that is required:

> *"Following the extraction, it is good to know that your body can begin to heal ... as it always does ... without the need for you to interfere ... you just have to follow the instructions that we give you ... and your body can do everything that is needed to heal ... . your body knows exactly how much blood is needed to make sure that the wound is clean ... and to fill in the socket so that it heals well ... consequently the bleeding will stop when there is just the right amount of blood in the socket."*

Imagery

Literal

Some patients may know, or would like to know, how the clotting mechanism works. A simple explanation such as the following will enable that person to use literal imagery to promote healthy, rapid healing.

> *"The blood flows to cleanse the wound, and to allow the raw material needed for healing to be where it is needed. Special cells called platelets gather at the edges, starting to form a dam, and a stringy substance called fibrin is produced, which creates a netting to trap the blood cells.*
>
> *The cells around the wound then begin to grow back over and around this fibrin scaffolding."*
>
> [This sort of explanation provides ample scope for imagery, both literal and figurative.]

Metaphorical

You can invite the patient to use imagery analogous to the healing process. For example, they might visualise themselves plastering over a crack in a wall or rebuilding a stone wall, or knitting, or might even visualise beavers constructing a dam. Given sufficient cues, most patients will be able to construct images applicable to themselves and their own lives.

Suggestions of altered physical sensation

Suggestions of cold around the damaged area (see glove analgesia, Chapter 25) might result in decreased blood flow and thus enhance the effects of other suggestions[13].

Ericksonian suggestion

Erickson uses the fact that the body is continually regulating the blood flow throughout the body[14]:

> *"In your present type of thinking, you do not believe that you could control the flow of blood; that you could cut down on bleeding. Yet you know that the utterance of one single word right now could bring a flush to the face ... and that is right, because your body has had lot of experience in controlling the flow of blood, and it is so easy and so simple ... and consider the way in which your body has had experience in turning pale at the thought of something terrifying, and consider the way your body has had many experiences in turning red under heat and white under cold.*

Your body has had a lot of experience; there is a tremendous wealth of actual physiological experience that warrants the expectation that one could build up a hypnotic situation to control capillary flow of blood. There is a wealth of knowledge that exists in your body, of which you are totally unaware, and that will manifest itself when given the right psychological and physiological stimulation."

The Management of Salivation

Hypnosis and imagery can have a profound effect upon the increase or decrease of the flow of saliva. Simply compare the dry mouth accompanying frightening imagery with the increased salivary flow we experience when we read an attractive menu.

Xerostomia – a dry mouth resulting from reduced or absent saliva flow – affects 1 in 4 people, and has the potential for causing much dental disease and discomfort. The condition is to some extent subjective in that there are many people who produce relatively low amounts of saliva without feeling too distressed, whereas others with higher levels feel the effects of a reduced flow very keenly[15].

Potential consequences of Xerostomia

1) Increased caries
2) Problems with dentures
3) Difficulties in eating dry food
4) Swollen salivary glands
5) Burning sensations and soreness
6) Ulceration
7) Increased susceptibility to infection

Before using any form of hypnotic intervention it is vital to diagnose the causes of the Xerostomia, and where necessary to treat with conventional methods. Causes can include infection, anxiety, medication, Sjogren's syndrome, AIDS/ HIV and irradiation. Artificial saliva, chewing gum and Pilocarpine can be of use, with more specific treatment of the particular condition[16].

Use of hypnosis

Managing anxiety and fear

As both anxiety and fear may be the cause of a dry mouth, hypnosis can be used to help the patient to cope with the problem (see Chapters 23 and 24).

Imagery to enhance the flow of saliva.

> *"... I'd like you to imagine a lemon ... a large juicy lemon ... that lovely yellow colour ... and you are just taking it out of the refrigerator ... and you feel the slight give in the skin as you hold it ... and you place it on a board ... and look at it ... and imagine the juiciness inside ... and you take a sharp kitchen knife ... and cut a slice out of that lemon ... and feel the resistance of the skin and the softness of the pulp as the juice squirts out ... and you take that slice and hold it near your nose ... and smell the sharp, tangy citrus smell of the lemon juice ... and you slowly put the slice of lemon in your mouth ... feeling the juice drip on your lips ... and crunch the lemon between your teeth and the bitter-sweet taste of that lemon juice ... squirts and flows into your mouth ... onto your tongue ... into your cheeks ... the floor of your mouth ... onto your palate ..."*

Metaphor

You might suggest the image of a stream gradually becoming a river. This image could also be used to alleviate any soreness: "as the water flows along ... cooling and soothing ... gentle and soft ... or even soothing the soreness".

Saliva reduction

Hypnosis can also be used to help reduce salivation – a very useful adjunct to operative dentistry.

Literal imagery

Invite the patient to imagine the glands gradually producing less saliva, and the tubes carrying the saliva to the mouth shrinking and contracting so that less saliva gets to the mouth.

Recall imagery

Invite the patient to remember a time when they had a very dry mouth, for instance when on holiday in beautiful sunshine. Note that it is important to emphasise that they access a happy, pleasant occasion so that the dry mouth has a comfortable connotation.

Metaphorical imagery

Suggest that the patient imagines turning down a tap or a valve of some sort that halts the flow of liquid, or that they imagine the sun's rays slowly evaporating the dew on the leaves of a plant or a flower.

Case history: Mandy – fissure sealing

The patient

Mandy, a sweet little seven-year-old, had attended regularly for dental check-ups since she was three and had never needed treatment. She thought it was great fun to sit in the dental chair and have her teeth examined. On this occasion an appointment had been made for her to have her permanent molars fissure-sealed. Unfortunately, Mandy had a large mobile tongue and produced excessive amounts of saliva (even though we were always careful not to make fissure seal appointments near to mealtimes!). Cotton wool rolls became soggy, access to the molars was virtually impossible, and Mandy became increasingly upset. With her mother's consent I asked Mandy if she'd like me to show her some magic and she responded enthusiastically.

Treatment plan

The plan was to create deep relaxation followed by "sleepy and dry" visualisation aimed at limiting saliva production and reducing tongue mobility.

Procedure

Induction and deepening was by balloon arm levitation followed by arm heaviness, to which Mandy responded excellently. My nurse at that time had a soft gentle voice, and at my request she read Mandy a short section from *The Wind in the Willows* by Kenneth Grahame, slowly and soothingly, with many pauses. As Mandy drifted deeply in trance, I seamlessly took over from my nurse and continued:

"... and it's so dreamy and drowsy and sleepy ... and your fingers can go to sleep and your toes can go to sleep ... and even your tongue can go to sleep ... just like the little animals and your best doll and your toys go to sleep every night ... and there's this lovely feeling in your lips and mouth and tongue ... just like when it's so lovely and hot and sunny ... and everything is so dry ... just like the warm sand when you go on holiday ... such a lovely feeling."

While I was speaking I was able to carry out fissure sealing in all four quadrants totally unimpeded by saliva or tongue movement. On my alerting Mandy, the nurse gave her a drink and we checked that all sensations were back to normal, at which the happy little girl ran back to her mother shouting: "He's done some magic!"

Outcome

Mandy remained a patient at the practice until she married at age twenty-three, and I'm happy to report that during all her time as a patient she never needed any fillings.

The Management of Aphthous Ulcers

Aphthous ulcers are among the most common oral lesions, affecting approximately 20% of the population. The ulcers generally occur on the non-keratinised oral mucosa, and can cause considerable pain and interference with eating, speaking and swallowing. Recurrent aphthous ulceration is classified as minor, major or herpetiform on the basis of the size and number of the ulcers.

There is no proven aetiology although immunological factors and emotional and physical stress have been implicated, with a high incidence occurring among students and military personnel[17]. Precipitating factors have been said to include trauma, stress, chemical irritants, hormones, and heredity[18]. Certain foods, including coffee, chocolate, potatoes, cheese, nuts, figs, citrus fruits and gluten-containing foods have also been implicated[19]. Deficiencies in iron, folate, and vitamin B-12 have also been noted in relation to the ulceration[20]. Interestingly, patients who have given up smoking report a higher incidence of aphthous ulceration, and it has been suggested that cigarette smoking prevents aphthous ulcers by causing increased keratinisation of the oral mucosa[21].

The primary goals of therapy are relief of pain, reduction of ulcer duration and restoration of normal oral function. Secondary goals include reduction in the frequency and severity of recurrences and maintenance of remission.

A number of infectious and autoimmune diseases, including Behçet's syndrome, Crohn's disease, lupus erythematosus and pemphigus vulgaris may result in oral ulceration, and a persistent oral ulcer could be carcinomatous. It is important, therefore, that when a patient presents with recurrent oral ulceration associated symptoms are elicited in order to eliminate further underlying pathology.

Hypnotic strategy

Often patients will tell you that they are seldom free of aphthous ulcers, and because stress is an aggravating feature patients will often have ulcers present when they attend for dental treatment. Hypnosis can be an effective tool in diminishing the stress and pain elements and in demonstrating to the patient that they have control over their oral mucosa. You can explain this to the patient before inviting them to use hypnosis in order to eradicate their problem. The hypnotic process will include imagery, self-analgesia, posthypnotic suggestion and self-hypnosis.

Procedure

Following induction and deepening, teach the patient self-hypnosis, focusing on imagery and feelings representing calmness, health and control. If the patient finds this imagery difficult to access, guide them into recognising the calm control they are showing at that moment with you in the surgery. When the patient has attained this, move on to teaching them glove analgesia (Chapter 25). Gain confirmation from the patient of the effectiveness of the glove analgesia by comparing the sensation of a needle prick or pinch into the skin of their "normal" hand and then their numbed hand. Strongly emphasise to them that they can now understand that they have control over their skin and the health of the skin lining their mouth, before continuing with the script below:

> *"... so now you can see that your skin is an organ of your body ... just as your heart and your stomach are parts of your body ... and you now know that you can actually control your skin ... and the skin on the inside of your mouth ... where you used to get ulcers ... so you now realise that as you can control the skin on the inside of your mouth ... just like you just showed us both how you can control the skin on the back of your hand ... you can keep the skin on your mouth strong and healthy and intact ... and this is what you'll do ... if at any time in the future you were to get that tingly feeling that used to come ... just before you used to get an ulcer ... then you take a breath ... and hold it for a few seconds ... and as you let the breath out remember how good you feel right now ... and say to yourself ... 'my skin is healthy' ... and all those feelings of calm control will just flow through your body ... and you'll probably find yourself quite surprised and really pleased with yourself ... as eventually you more or less forget that you ever used to get ulcers ..."* [Here introduce ego-strengthening and forward pacing to a future time when ulcers are no longer a problem.]

Advise the patient to use self-hypnosis every day with emphasis on calmness, health and control, and with a mantra such as "my skin is healthy" flowing through their mind.

Case history: Stephen – recurrent aphthous ulceration

> *The patient*
> Stephen was a 27-year-old post-graduate university student and had been a dental patient at the practice since childhood, never having required any conservation treatment.

Since the age of 16 he had been affected by extremely painful, large and discrete aphthous ulcers virtually every time I saw him. The ulcers were typically on the lateral borders of his tongue and on his buccal mucosa at occlusal level. Palliative treatment had included various topical corticosteroids and anti-inflammatory preparations and lozenges, and I had referred him to his GP who had found no underlying pathology.

I explained to Stephen that sometimes our immune system can work against us, and possibly that was what was wrong in this case. Reframing this, I said that this was good news because his immune system must be powerful, and therefore through hypnosis we would train it to work *for* him rather than *against* him. Stephen was enthusiastic so we made an immediate start.

Procedure

Stephen responded well to eye-roll induction, and deepening by imagery incorporating a sense of control and success was effective. (Stephen later told me that his image was of seeing his name on the notice board when he achieved a First in his Finals.) I taught Stephen how to intensify the sounds, sights and feelings of the image to the extent of drowning out my voice, and then quietly reiterated the important role of the immune system and that he could now start to take control of his mouth. Before alerting Stephen I gave him instruction in regular 10-second self-hypnosis episodes, to incorporate a clenched fist anchor coupled with a mantra: "*I'm in control.*"

The following week I introduced Stephen to glove analgesia (see Chapter 25) and used that achievement to reinforce the previous session's suggestions of control. I followed this by ego-strengthening based upon his Degree and his performance with me. I also instructed him in forward pacing to a time when he realised that he no longer had any ulcers, and also strongly suggested that he continue with his self-hypnosis.

Outcome

This all took place twenty years ago and regular Christmas cards carry the message that Stephen has had literally no aphthous ulcers from the time of the first session.

References

1. Coué E. Self-Mastery Through Conscious Autosuggestion. Whitefish, MT: Kessinger Publishing, 1977.
2. Hartland J. Medical and Dental Hypnosis. London: Baillière Tindall, 1966.
3. Freud S. The Ego and the Id. London: Hogarth Press, 1923.
4. Heap M, Aravind KK. Hartland's Medical and Dental Hypnosis. London: Churchill Livingstone, 2002.
5. Stanton HE. Adorning the clenched fist technique. Contemporary Hypnosis 1997;14:189–94.
6. Cheek DB, Cron LML. Clinical Hypnotherapy. New York: Grune and Statton, 1968.
7. Bandler R, Grinder J. The Structure of Magic. Palo Alto, CA: Science and Behavior Books, 1975.
8. Stein C. Clenched-fist as a hypnobehavioral procedure. Am J Clin Hypn 1963;2:113–19.
9. Schultz JH, Luthe W. Autogenic training: A Psychophysiologic Approach in Psychotherapy. New York: Grune and Stratton, 1959.
10. Rossi EL. The Psychobiology of Mind-Body Healing. New York: W. W. Norton & Company, 1986.
11. Hopkins B, Jordan J, Lundy RM. The effects of hypnosis and of imagery on bleeding time: a brief communication. Int J Clin Exp Hyp 1991;139:34–9.
12. Enquist B, von Konow L, Bystedt H. Pre- and perioperative suggestion in maxillofacial surgery: effects on blood loss and recovery. Int J Clin Exp Hyp 1995;43: 284–94.
13. Bishay EG, Lee C. Studies of the effects of hypnoanesthesia on regional blood flow by transcutaneous oxygen monitoring. Am J Clin Hypn 1984;27(1): 64–9.
14. Erickson M. Healing in Hypnosis Vol. 1. New York: Irvington, 1983.
15. Billings R. Studies on the prevalence of xerostomia. Preliminary results. Caries Research 1989;23: Abstr. 124(35th ORCA congress).
16. Thornhill M. Xerostomia: Care and Management. London: Wrigley, 2004.
17. Fischman SL. Oral ulcerations. Semin Dermatol 1994;Jun. 13(2):74–7.
18. Rodu B, Mattingly G. Oral mucosal ulcers: diagnosis and management. J Am Dent Assoc 1992;Oct. 123(10):83–6.
19. Petersen MJ, Baughman RA. Recurrent aphthous stomatitis: primary care management. Nurse Pract 1996;May 21(5):36–40.
20. Schneider LC, Schneider AE. Diagnosis of oral ulcers. Mt Sinai J Med 1998;Oct.–Nov. 65(5–6):383–7.
21. Grady D, Emster V, Stillman I, Greenspan J. Oral Surg Oral Med O 1992;Oct. 74(4):463–5.

21

Psychodynamic Therapy

Hypnosis can be used as an adjunct to many different types of psychological therapy, and has been shown to increase the effectiveness of a range of recognised treatments. The process of change can be powerfully facilitated by the patient's enhanced relaxation, imagery and affect, coupled with their ability to "opt out" and rapidly restore equilibrium when necessary.

In this chapter we will briefly explain the differences and similarities of some recognised therapeutic approaches, and focus upon psychodynamic therapy. Some useful hypnotic techniques are based on concepts described by Sigmund Freud and the psychoanalytical school, and these include abreaction, affect bridge, ideomotor signalling, regression and approaches that use the metaphor of the unconscious or subconscious mind.

An overview of some psychotherapeutic approaches

Most of the references to the use of hypnosis in dentistry that you will find in this book will relate broadly to humanistic and cognitive-behavioural psychotherapeutic processes. In assuming that you will be using hypnosis as an adjunct to your normal skills in order to facilitate dental practice as rapidly, easily and comfortably as possible for both the patient and yourself, we will be concentrating upon these largely "here and now" approaches.

Humanistic approach

Humanistic psychotherapy, derived from the work of Carl Rogers[1], is based on precepts that we feel should be ever present in our relationship with patients. Rogers' core principles are of unconditional positive regard, genuineness and empathic understanding. This approach touches upon all aspects of communication and relationships with patients (see Chapter 3, 4 and 6), and forms part of the rapport and trust-building intrinsic to all aspects of clinical hypnosis.

Behavioural approach

The behaviour therapies have developed to a large extent from the workings of Pavlov, Watson, Skinner and others (see Chapter 24), and in essence are a form of training. A principle is that the patient does not need to understand why he behaves in a certain way, the central issue being that his responses to reward and reinforcement (for example, through ego-strengthening) serve to change the unwanted behaviour.

For example, a child who behaves well at the dentist may be given a sticker.

Cognitive-behavioural approach

Cognitive-behavioural therapies assume that the individual's maladaptive behaviour and negative emotions are a result of maladaptive thinking patterns[2]. The aim of therapy is to correct this by focusing on altering the patient's thoughts and assumptions. In other words, the engagement of the patient's cognition means that thoughtful awareness becomes involved and there is some mental processing of the ensuing behaviour.

The approach to the smoker might be: "… I wonder if you've thought about the amount of damage that smoking can do to your mouth and your teeth as well as your general health … would you like to work with me to do something about it …?"

Psychodynamic approach

Psychodynamic therapy is aimed at helping the individual to understand the roots of their emotional distress, and the possibly *unconscious* factors that drive their behaviour. Hypnosis, largely through the relaxation of the patient's normal defences, allows them to "regress" to earlier life experiences, often experiencing "abreaction" and "affect bridge" responses.

The focus for the smoker: "… I wonder what it is that gives you the need to smoke … where that unconscious urge comes from … maybe we can take a look at that so that you can find out how you might change …"

Language and concepts

"Conscious" and "unconscious"

In this section we will be using such concepts as *conscious* and *unconscious*, and to avoid any ambiguity it is important to put these words into the context within which we will be using them. For this purpose we shall use a model in which the *conscious mind* is what we are aware of at any particular moment, our present perceptions, memories, thoughts, fantasies and feelings.

Working closely with the conscious mind is the *preconscious*, our "available memory", comprising memories we are not at the moment thinking about but that can easily be brought to mind. The preconscious is just below the surface but not available unless we search for it. Information such as our telephone number, some childhood memories or the name of our best childhood friend is stored in the preconscious.

By far the largest part in this model is the *unconscious*. This includes all the things that are not easily available to awareness. Freud believed that the greater part of what we experience in our lives, the underlying emotions, beliefs, feelings and impulses, is not accessible to us at a conscious level, and that the part that drives our feelings and behaviour is buried in our unconscious.

The relation of this to ideomotor signalling

When we use ideomotor signalling we can introduce the idea by suggesting to the patient that they are simply allowing their "unconscious mind" to answer by flickering a finger in much the same way as they might unconsciously nod or shake their head. Some therapist may use the phrase "that part at the back of your mind" to describe the unconscious part.

For practical purposes it is probably better to think in terms of an ideomotor signal taking place *without conscious volition* – a sort of *impromptu* and *spontaneous* answer. Like many hypnotic procedures, it might be seen as a metaphor indicating that the patient is prepared to trust the therapist and to explore their problem with him. In doing this the patient is also implicitly showing their willingness to deepen their trance.

How might all this relate to memory?

We do not intend in this book to examine in depth the theories and controversies that surround such concepts as *repressed* and *false* memories. (Readers who wish to study the relation between hypnosis and such phenomena are advised to read *Hartland's Medical and Dental Hypnosis*[3], pp. 201–215.)

However, there are certain points relevant to the practical use of hypnosis in uncovering techniques and psychodynamic therapy that we will now examine.

Memories retrieved during hypnosis are not necessarily accurate. Hypnosis and ideomotor responses are not lie detectors. Through empathy the patient will feel safe and may disclose true memories that they had previously withheld. Because hypnosis also enhances the ability to fantasise, and these fantasies can seem real to the patient, memories can assume a sense of certainty in the patient's mind. Coupled with this may be the patient's misplaced expectation of hypnosis, and a belief that through it they can accurately "relive" earlier experiences. Consequently it is important that you disabuse the patient of the expectation that they will recover "the truth" about a deep-seated problem, at the same time reassuring them that material that may come to light in hypnosis can be helpful in the resolution of their problem, and that they can feel safe in letting themselves express the emotions accompanying such memories.

Abreaction and Affect Bridge

Abreaction

An abreaction is an intense emotional release or discharge. It can arise with or without hypnosis, and you have probably already experienced this with some patients. Abreaction in hypnosis occurs when the patient, generally involuntarily, relives a painful experience. Superficially at least the experience recalled may not seem to be appropriate to the patient's current experience, but the *affect* always is. It is claimed that the emotional content of the memory evoked has been *repressed* because consciously that experience was too unpleasant to face up to, and it may be helpful to explain this to the patient. The emotion generated may be quite mild and transient, or so powerful that it may seem as though the patient is actually reliving the experience.

Although the emotions expressed may represent the emotions of a child and the recall may be that of a childhood incident, the responses will actually be those of the here and now adult and may be an unconscious reinterpretation of the child's feelings (see Martin Orne, page 12).

Case history: Wendy – behind every adult is a child

> *The patient*
> Wendy, a well-dressed and well-spoken young woman, arrived at the surgery in a very distressed state having been given an emergency appointment to deal with a broken tooth. She was white-faced, crying and trembling, and said that the thought of coming to a dental surgery must have triggered off this *"state of collapse".*
>
> Despite her distress and weeping, rapport was established and she allowed me to examine the tooth and apply a temporary dressing.

I was interested to see that although her dentition was excellent and well cared for she had a denture replacing *321/123*. During the treatment Wendy remained extremely tense, struggling to maintain her composure.

Treatment plan

At her request an appointment was made with the aim of taking her through a hypno-desensitisation programme in order that she might deal with the necessary local anaesthetic and restoration more comfortably.

Procedure

At her appointment two weeks later, Wendy was much more composed and entered hypnosis readily following an eye-roll induction. Almost immediately she underwent an intense abreaction, screaming, sobbing and shaking her head and body, all the time apparently in deep trance with her eyes closed. My nurse and I calmed her and let her cry until after about 10 minutes she appeared to relax deeply into hypnosis. I reassured her of her well-being here and now and gave her the suggestion that:

> *"... I don't know what triggered that off, but maybe deep in your unconscious mind you do know ... and soon, but before you become alert again ... you can allow that memory to go back where it was ... deep in your unconscious as it was before ... only bringing into your consciousness anything that you feel strong enough and able to deal with here and now as the adult that you now are ... and I don't need to know any of this ... but if there's anything you feel you* do *want to tell me then you can do so ... and if you wish to we can use that knowledge to help you to move forward ..."*

When Wendy was alerted, she was shaken but appeared relieved to have dealt with her thoughts, and though quietly sobbing told me the following story.

Five years previously she had lived with a partner who during their time together had been diagnosed as schizophrenic. One night he had violently beaten her up, smashing her anterior teeth. She had been rushed to hospital and given a general anaesthetic, and the remaining roots had been extracted. She told me that the greatest horror had been half-waking as the operation was being completed and having an "out of body experience" of looking down on herself as though seeing a corpse with a toothless open mouth pouring with blood. The horror of this had haunted her and had shot into her mind as the hypnosis in my dental chair began.

I explained that, if she wanted, we could use hypnosis to help her deal with this terrible memory, and she expressed eagerness to do so. I told her that the experience would possibly be quite emotional but that we would first establish a "safe place" to which she could retreat if the emotions were too overpowering. I assured her that she was safe and secure here and now, and to emphasise this we established an anchor of my hand on her right shoulder.

Using an affect bridge, Wendy regressed once again to the memory and emotions of that night, and again abreacted strongly, but this time with the knowledge that she could opt out if things became unbearable, and between us, using a TV video technique, we laid that demon to rest.

On alerting and reassurances, Wendy said, *"I'm sure there's more ... something else."*

We repeated the process and Wendy abreacted much more powerfully than she had done the previous time, this time crying out in a childlike voice. Again we worked through the abreaction until Wendy felt a sense of completion. On alerting she told me the following.

At about the age of six she had been taken to the dentist to have a tooth out. She had no idea what to expect. She recalled a "large, unfriendly" nurse grabbing her hand and pulling her away from her mother and into the surgery where she was "roughly plonked down into this big chair". The dentist, whom she described as "frowning, cold and silent", then gave her what she now knows was an injection. She did not recall this as being painful. The dentist and nurse then ignored her and were chatting to each other in the corner of the room while this frightening thing happened.

"My face started going funny, as though it was dead, as though it was dropping off. It was so scary and I started to cry. And no one took any notice. Eventually the nurse said, 'Don't be such a baby,' and the dentist just scowled and just pulled my tooth out. I was really scared but I don't remember it hurting. I think the main thing was that no one seemed to care. I felt so alone and frightened."

Following reassurances, Wendy was happy to enter hypnosis again, and on my suggestion took the role of caring mother, speaking out aloud and giving love and necessary support to the little girl. After about 10 minutes Wendy smiled through her tears and said, *"That feels so good. Everything's OK now."*

Since then Wendy has been a model patient, and her experience is a constant reminder to me of the importance of gentleness and caring, particularly when working with child patients.

Managing abreaction

When a powerful abreaction appears from out of the blue it can be very distressing for both patient and therapist as there is often no warning or obvious reason for the sudden release. Your major role is to be a calm, quiet and reassuring recipient of the patient's outpourings, making no attempt to intervene other than in "being there" for the patient. Often following the abreaction the patient will be tired and confused and will value the emotional let-up. At this stage you may give general reassurance and guide the patient into deep relaxation. You can then give ego-strengthening suggestions, in essence congratulating the patient on facing and coming through such a difficult experience, and preparing the ground for successful future work.

A helpful way of describing abreaction to a patient is to use the metaphor of a pressure cooker. Events in life can build up into an emotional pressure and sometimes we can be frightened that the pressure is so great it will explode. By releasing some of that pressure bit by bit in a safe environment, as with the valve on a pressure cooker, it can be released in manageable amounts so that we remain safe and in control.

Potentially abreaction, although initially upsetting, is beneficial, allowing some desensitisation of the distressing emotions or giving the patient greater insight into their experiences. Their trust in exposing themselves to you, and the recognition that you are empathic, caring and non-judgemental will strengthen rapport and thus facilitate future treatment. The main risk, however, is that the experience does not bring relief but further traumatises the patient, increasing their perception that dentistry is a situation of emotional trauma.

If you feel that the abreaction is not going to bring about some relief, then it is necessary to help the patient leave the experience behind by stressing that that traumatic experience is in the past, and congratulating them on having survived it to be here now, and having the courage to deal with it.

When the patient has been alerted you may gently invite them to tell you about it, always giving them the option of not so doing. It may be that as a result of the issues raised during that experience the patient may need to revisit the material before proceeding with the original treatment plan. However, often this release of emotion is all that is required and may in itself be therapeutic, and at the next appointment you might continue with their dental treatment as normal.

Although it is not within the scope of this book to discuss in detail the various techniques used hypnotically to manage abreaction, it is worth a brief mention of the options available.

Transactional technique

When a memory of a childhood incident is cited by the patient, within hypnosis you might suggest that the now adult patient can comfort the then child appropriately:

> "... I wonder what you'd like to say and do for that little girl right now ... what it would take to make her feel alright again ... because you, as an adult ... with all the wisdom and experience ... and your deep knowledge of that little girl ... know exactly what she needs ... so why don't you comfort her and tell her the things that'll make her feel better ..."

Although this hypnotic acting out may bring tears, this tends to bring comfort and a sense of completion to the patient.

Wolberg's theatre technique (and TV update)

Here, by means of hypnotic visualisation of either a theatre or a TV video player, the patient is encouraged to run through the scene as though seeing it acted out, and subsequently, as director, to alter the action to create a more acceptable and comfortable action and completion[4].

Through this the patient is able to achieve a sense of dissociation from the trauma and of control over the situation, and at the same time can carry out a form of forward pacing.

Case history: James – injection panic

The patient

James was a pleasant young man who became acutely anxious whenever he needed an injection. He would panic and feel as though he had to get away, and had often fainted at some time during the procedure.

He was a very fit, healthy person, with good oral hygiene, but needed two restorations replacing. This filled him with dread and also made him feel embarrassed and annoyed with himself. During the history-taking, he explained that as a small child he sometimes travelled with his mother, who was a district nurse, to visit patients. Part of her work involved taking blood and giving injections.

Treatment plan

After further discussion, we decided to use regression to identify and resolve any experiences which were responsible for his current situation.

Procedure

Induction was by simple "eye roll" and was followed by progressive relaxation. At this stage ego-strengthening suggestions were given, and James was taught self-hypnosis. He was then given a post-hypnotic suggestion that he would go easily and quickly into hypnosis at later visits.

The second session again began with an eye-roll induction followed by progressive relaxation, and an ideomotor response was established.

I told James that he would hear my voice very clearly, and recognise it as belonging to someone friendly, helpful and supportive, wherever he felt that he was [*Erickson*].

Next, I asked him to imagine as vividly as possible an occasion when he felt really good, in control, having a sense of achievement and being very confident. When he signalled that he had reached this, I pressed firmly on his shoulder, with the instruction that every time he felt that same pressure in that area he would feel all those same good, positive feelings [*anchoring*].

I then asked James to imagine himself in a cinema, about to watch a film of his life. He would have total control over that film, in that he could view whatever section he liked, at any time, in any way. Firstly, he was asked to view a happy scene from his past, and then to set up the film to just before an event that would be relevant to his current situation.

As the film progressed I gave reassuring suggestions, and triggered the anchor. I advised James that he could then step into the film, to offer support, reassurance and comfort to that younger self; he could allow all those positive feelings to pass over to that younger self, and I explained that he need not be as frightened or as upset about that situation again. After a signal confirming that he had spent sufficient time doing all this, I asked him to let the film run forward to some time in the future, and to experience as vividly as possible, how well he would deal with similar situations in the future. I then invited him to allow the film to go to any other events that could have relevance to the present, but he decided that there was nothing else to review.

Outcome

On alerting, James told me that he had had a vivid recollection of an old caravan in the Dales, where his mother would treat patients. He was four years old, and was very receptive to the feelings such as anxiety and pain shown by many of the patients, and his mother was so used to her job that she never realised the effect it was having on her little boy. James felt alone in the corner of the caravan thinking that it could well be his turn next, and the thought of seeing his own blood and feeling like the other people made him feel as if he had to escape, but was unable to do so.

Following my reassurances and ego-strengthening suggestions, James said that he felt a lot more comfortable about the thought of having an injection, and that it all seemed less threatening.

One week later, James attended for the restorations. Although he appeared a little tense and he reported afterwards that he felt his heart beat a little faster, he felt it was a vast improvement on his previous experiences, and he did not feel in the least bit faint.

Since then, James has been able to watch TV programmes including invasive procedures, which previously would have caused him great distress, and subsequent dental visits have been uneventful.

Affect bridge

Affect bridge, described by Watkins[5], is a process by which the patient accesses previous memories by focusing on an emotional or physical feeling that they are experiencing in the present, and using that feeling as a link to a previous event where that same feeling occurred. Although this experience can occur without hypnosis, in hypnosis it will tend to be more vivid and intense and can be used therapeutically, and care needs to be taken to help the patient through the event without undue distress.

Explanation

A helpful way of describing affect bridge to a patient may be to use the analogy of a train coming to a gentle stop. Immediately after the engine comes to a halt the first wagon clangs into it, then the second clangs into the buffers of the first, and so on right the way down the train. In the same way our emotional response to a perceived trauma can trigger off a sequence of reverberation back through time, triggering off an emotional recall of events that in any *symbolic* way relate to the present trauma. It is important to note that the actual events may not appear similar, but the *affect*, the emotional response, is the trigger. Thus a feeling of fear might cause emotional recall of a whole variety of times of fear across a whole spectrum of experience.

The use of affect bridge regression

There will be times when a patient tells you that there is some aspect of treatment that they simply cannot tolerate. Other patients characteristically at some point during dental treatment might suddenly jerk their head away, or push your hands away and/or experience a severe abreaction. There will be many occasions where you and the patient together can rationalise their sudden panic, identify the cause and negotiate ways of managing the problem.

Where the patient's problem seems intractable by simple hypnotic suggestion and behavioural strategies, affect bridge regression may be a treatment of choice.

Procedure

Firstly explain to the patient what affect bridge work entails, possibly using the train metaphor described earlier. Reassure them that although there may be times during the work that they find upsetting, they will remain safe and secure throughout and you will be with them as a source of strength and support. Reassure them that before alerting them you will make sure that they are fully integrated with "here and now", and that they are likely to feel much happier about themselves and dental treatment in the future.

Procedure for affect bridge

When the patient has agreed to the use of hypnosis, carry out induction and deepening.

Set up an ideomotor signal response and a positive anchor (for affect bridge, a shoulder anchor is the method of choice).

Ask the patient to recall a recent time when they experienced that particular sensation and encourage them to express the emotion that the recall evokes.

Intensify these feelings until the patient is experiencing them as deeply as is possible for them at that time, while letting the underlying situation itself fade away.

Suggest that the patient uses the feelings to take themselves back to any previous time they have experienced these same feelings.

At this stage the patient may emote quite powerfully and it is important that you are ready to offer comfort and support as this process occurs. At the same time give appropriate suggestions or reframes to promote resolution of the problem.

When the patient seems to have found a sense of resolution invite them to review any other incidents that they feel are relevant, and encourage resolution.

Gain feedback from the patient on their new current feelings about the past, and their attitude towards continuing with dental treatment.

Give further performance-based ego-strengthening suggestions and reassurance.

On alerting, give the patient the option of describing their experience, check out their feelings about the experience and the resolution of their problem, and invite them to continue with their dental treatment either straight away or at a future appointment.

Case history: Julie – the use of affect bridge regression

The patient

Julie was a 35-year-old woman, and this was her first visit to the practice. She had no trace of nerves and sat down readily in the dental chair for her inspection. I started tilting the chair and suddenly, at about the halfway point, Julie went very pale, jerked her hands up to her mouth and started crying hysterically. I immediately righted the chair and my nurse and I soothed and supported Julie until she regained her composure. She apologised, said she was really ashamed and that she didn't know what had come over her, but as the chair had gone back she had just freaked out.

Following discussion, her examination was completed with the chair in the upright position and an appointment made for Julie to return for hypnosis to be used to facilitate her necessary dental conservation.

Treatment plan

My aim was to use hypnotic relaxation coupled to desensitisation, possibly using the image of a beach lounger as we incrementally tilted the chair backwards. This was explained to Julie and she said that she would be happy to do this.

Procedure

Eye-roll induction was followed by progressive muscular relaxation and a beach image, an ideomotor response was established and Julie became extremely deeply relaxed. With appropriate suggestions, I slowly and with pauses tilted the chair. Again at the halfway point Julie abreacted violently, screaming hysterically, jerking her head and body and shrieking *"no, no, no!"*. My nurse and I too were shocked, and we calmed her as I re-raised the chair and allowed her once again to regain her composure.

Following further discussion, explanation and reassurance, we decided to use affect bridge technique together with a shoulder anchor to attempt to deal with Julie's problem. I told Julie that she would be able to talk to me if she wished, and that my hand on her shoulder would protect her against too much distress.

With Julie in hypnosis I suggested: *"... you go back to a few minutes ago ... and relive as much as you feel you can what you were feeling then ... and go as far as you feel you can ... knowing that you will always be safe here"* [*rehearsing the shoulder anchor*]. Julie again abreacted, but in a more controlled way. I continued:

"... I don't know what triggered that off, but maybe deep in your unconscious mind you do. Are you prepared to go into your unconscious mind to find out what is going on? [Julie signalled affirmation] *Great. So now go deep in your unconscious and let those feelings take you to where they come from ... and any time you want to stop, your 'no' finger will let me know ..."*

Julie abreacted as before, but somehow seemed to be more in control. Remaining in hypnosis, and through her distress and tears, she told me how, when she was a child of eight, the doctor had removed her tonsils without anaesthetic as she lay on the kitchen table. I let her work through the emotions and as she slowly regained control, though still in hypnosis, I used the transactional model as described in the case of "Wendy" (above) so that Julie could reintegrate the memory with the surviving and grown-up person she had become. When she signalled that she was ready I alerted her. She then told me the story again, adding that it was a "real" memory and something that cropped up in family conversations, often in almost joking fashion, but she hadn't realised how much pain was still involved within the memory.

Outcome

At Julie's request then we reverted to the original plan of desensitisation with beach lounger imagery. After initial trepidation Julie responded well and from then on we had no further problems with her treatment in the normal supine position.

Discussion

Rossi[6] uses the term "state-dependent learning" to describe that:

"Inasmuch as experience arises from the binding or coupling of a particular state or level of arousal with a particular symbolic interpretation of that arousal, experience is state bound."

In Julie's case it could be argued that at a rational level she remembered the trauma she had experienced as that child, but only when she was placed in a symbolic or analogous situation, supine and about to suffer an assault in her mouth, was the bonded level of arousal revivified, giving rise to her "emotional memory" and thus the abreaction.

23

Pain, Fear and Anxiety

It is impossible to separate the sensation of pain from the emotion of fear. A feeling of fear, anxiety and apprehension will inevitably accentuate the patient's perception of pain. Equally, pain experienced at the dental surgery will inevitably lead to increased fear and anxiety at the prospect of further visits.

Consequently any strategies that reduce either the fear or the pain that a patient associates with dentistry will interact. Within this chapter we will begin by examining pain and fear separately and then concentrate upon their unavoidable intimate connection.

Pain

While there can be no substitute for clinical excellence, pain management lies at the core of very much of the practical work that we do. Indeed many patients will choose their dentist on the recommendation of a friend who says "I didn't feel a thing".

It is possible to achieve excellent results with minimum discomfort, and there can be little doubt that it is far easier to do good dentistry on a relaxed pain-free patient than upon someone who is nervous and who reacts strongly to even the slightest stimulus.

The control and relief of pain is one of the most useful and rewarding aspects of hypnosis in clinical practice. The perception of pain is the outcome of a complex combination of many diverse factors.

Note the word "perception"; pain is a consequence of what the patient *perceives it to be* rather than a simple matter of stimulus–response.

Much of the anxiety surrounding dentistry is based upon fear of procedural pain, particularly that accompanying injections and fillings[7].

Categories of pain

There are three major categories of pain that overlap, and our primary concern as dentists who incorporate hypnosis within our work is procedural pain.

Acute pain
Acute pain is a symptom that is biologically useful and recognised as having a "real" cause. It is generally self-limiting and its management and relief are usually possible. It can be associated with anxiety and distress, sometimes as acute as the pain itself. In dental terms its most common presentation is toothache.

Chronic pain
The pain itself is a disease having no biological usefulness, and relief is often challenging if not impossible. The prolonged experience of pain may cause severe depression, have a deleterious effect on heart and kidneys, disturb gastric and colonic processes, and upset heart regularity and blood pressure. The price of such pain in terms of reduced efficiency at work and impact upon all aspects of life is hard to measure.

Procedural pain
Procedural pain is a major issue as much of our professional life is spent in carrying out procedures that have the potential to cause pain and distress. Inevitably the responsibility of being perceived as the purveyor of pain can result in negative effects upon dentists' self-image and ultimately upon their health, a powerful motivation for the introduction of hypnosis into dental practice[8].

Definition of pain

There are innumerable definitions of pain, and Hart's[9] includes the multiplicity of factors affecting the patient's perception:
> *"... a multi-dimensional psychobiosocial experience including real sensory input, emotional factors (e.g. suffering, fear, expectation, mood, anxiety, tension, suggestion, memory and motivation), and social components (e.g. cultural and environmental consequences)."*

In practical terms pain might also be described as:
> *"What the patient says hurts." (the Authors, 2006)*

Dimensions of pain

When a pain stimulus occurs and activates the receptor system, it enters an active nervous system that is already primed by such factors as past experience, cultural learning, anxiety and present meaning of the pain. Consequently the pain experience is a dynamic process that involves continuous interaction between complex ascending and descending systems.

The pain response is complex and includes the *sensory-discriminative*, the *motivational-affective* and the *cognitive-evaluative* components. So in using hypnosis within pain management we are dealing with the combination of sensation, and the emotional suffering that goes with it and the person's evaluation of its meaning. Each system will influence the other two, so that the pain response is dynamic rather than static and is self-perpetuating, giving rise to a feedback spiral. Specific hypnotic techniques are applicable to all of these components and will be described in the next part of the book.

Many strategies are superimposed upon one another in hypnotic pain reduction. Identifying a patient's cognitive style and assumptions about the pain will suggest the potential route for any hypnotic suggestions.

Often a patient's fear might seem irrational, and the desperate lengths that some sufferers will go to in order to avoid a visit to the dentist might appear to be painful and dangerous. Press reports give examples of people extracting their own teeth at home with pliers, such is their fear of visiting a dentist. For many of us the time and energy spent in dealing with patients' fears and anxieties can be frustrating and debilitating, and can in extreme cases give rise to fatigue and burn-out.

Fear

Despite the huge technological advances in dentistry, and the relative comfort that patients can now enjoy, dental fear and anxiety remain a serious problem for many people. Dental anxiety is common worldwide, with figures for its prevalence varying between 10% and 15%[10-12]. The latest adult dental health survey reported that about a third of dentate adults definitely agreed that they always felt anxious about going to the dentist[13].

Fear and anxiety are part of the normal human experience and all of us have the potential for a phobic response. However, as long as we do not have to face or experience the object of our phobia there is little problem. For example, a city dweller with a phobia of sharks is unlikely to be confronted by one, and a person with acrophobia can usually avoid climbing mountains. In his novel 1984, George Orwell introduced the concept of "Room 101" within which lurked each individual's worst thing in the world: "There are occasions when a human being will stand out against pain, even to the point of death. But for everyone there is something unendurable – something that cannot be contemplated."[14]

So within dentistry the object of the phobia must be confronted when it becomes necessary for a dentally phobic patient to attend for treatment. For many people avoidance is the "easy" option, but possibly, after twenty years of relatively comfortable avoidance of dentistry, a dental phobic awakes one morning with excruciating toothache, the severity of the pain overcomes the phobia, and the terrified patient arrives at the surgery.

This can put immense pressure upon a dentist and his staff, and in many circumstances hypnosis can play a major role in the management of the situation.

Expectation plays a central role in pain perception. In the dental setting pain is expected, and can be produced by anxiety. Pain and anxiety have a "chicken and egg" relationship – a low pain threshold and dental phobia are linked, but distinguishing between chicken and egg as a starting point can prove difficult[15].

What is fear?

Fear is a normal and necessary response to danger and is essential for our defence, safety and survival. Generally the sequence of events within the experience of fear is cognition of a perceived threat instantly followed by a reflex response of the autonomic nervous system, giving rise to a range of physical changes, commonly referred to as "the fight or flight" response. In modern times, even though many of our perceived threats are of a psychological nature the fight or flight response still occurs, and by its very nature is often more of an impediment than a help in handling the feared situation.

The fear response is characterised by an instantaneous action of the sympathetic nervous system to a perceived danger. As a result of this the heart rate becomes rapid and breathing accelerates in order to maximise the passage of oxygen through the lungs to the blood stream, and to pump the oxygenated blood to the muscles of the limbs. As a consequence the limbs will often feel weak and shaky. This diversion of blood away from the viscera will often result in unpleasant sensations within the abdomen, and may lead to a desire for the individual to defecate, urinate or vomit.

Because of diversion of blood away from the head region, the fearful patient may appear pale faced and in a cold sweat, and his short-term memory may be impaired, giving rise to confusion. The net result is often that the feedback of these unpleasant feelings to the individual becomes in itself an object of fear, and thus a spiral is set up possibly leading to a "panic attack".

Anxiety

There are many similarities between anxiety and fear, but the context and intensity may differ. Although physiologically the same mechanisms operate, while fear is normally related to a specific object or situation, anxiety tends to relate to the mental processing of such a situation, and so is frequently experienced when the individual is not actually in the presence of the stimulus. Indeed, anxiety occurs in many people for no apparent reason, and this in turn might give rise to a self-perpetuating spiral of anxiety about the anxiety.

Anxiety, like fear, has a positive element, designed to protect the individual and to enhance that individual's performance and coping ability. For example, anxiety before an examination may provide a stimulus for study and for alertness. However, too great a degree of anxiety in advance of the examination might result in a lack of sleep and a confused mind; an obvious disadvantage.

It is possible to define three categories of the anxiety experience.

- First there is the "normal" anxiety that occurs before an important event such as an interview or presentation, which overall is controllable and can be beneficial to performance.
- Second there is the "phobic anxiety" relating to an object or situation that is perceived, rationally or irrationally, as threatening. Dental anxiety would fall into this category.
- Third is "free-floating anxiety" in which the individual has the psychological and physical feelings described, but no reason is apparent to him.

So although both fear and anxiety produce physiological changes that are disturbing and unpleasant to the individual, neither is an "all or nothing" response, and there is a great variation in the intensity of the feelings experienced.

Phobia

A phobia is profound fear and anxiety, usually, but not necessarily, of a specific perceived threat or situation, the severity of which is so unpleasant as to be disabling. Dental phobia is an exaggerated fear of dentists and dental procedures. Although phobia is defined as an "irrational" fear', in the context of dentistry many sufferers will relate the phobia to an earlier bad experience, and thus the phobia might fall into the category of a learned conditioned response[16]. Additional subcategories could be "fear of dentists" and a phobia of specific procedures, such as extractions or objects such as needles. In many instances anticipation of, or confrontation with, the feared object or situation, may precipitate a panic attack.

For virtually all patients with phobia the state is self-perpetuating. In other words the fear of a phobic attack can be so severe that it precipitates the attack. People when asked what they are most fearful of will say "I don't want to make a scene", "I think I might faint", "I think I'm going to die".

Characteristically, the sufferer will endure the phobic situation with intense anxiety and distress, or will avoid the situation by not visiting the dentist. A dentist once said that he was not troubled by dental phobics because they never turned up!

For adults the avoidance and anxious anticipation of distress in the feared situation(s) can significantly interfere with the person's life, and there may often be marked distress, shame and guilt about having the phobia. In children, the anxiety is often expressed by crying, tantrums, freezing, or clinging.

Panic attack

A panic attack is defined as the sudden onset of an period of *intense* fear or discomfort, and will characteristically include a number of the physical and psychological symptoms described in Table 23.1.

Table 23.1 **Symptoms of a panic attack**

Physical symptoms	Psychological symptoms
• trembling, shortness of breath and tightness across the chest • sweating and palpitations, dizziness or light-headedness, nausea or abdominal discomfort • tingling and pins and needles • hot flushes or chills	• a sense of unreality • a fear of losing control • a fear of going mad or "making a fool of myself" • a fear of fainting or dying • a feeling of iminent danger and a need to escape

Learning and unlearning fear and anxiety

Almost all behaviour, including the fearful patient's feelings about dental treatment, is a *learned* response to a situation. The natural corollary of this is that the role of hypnosis in behaviour management is to help the patient to *unlearn* their current maladaptive behaviour and learn a new, successful behaviour. We shall now look at three familiar learning principles.

Classical conditioning

Ivan Pavlov[17] introduced the concept of *classical conditioning* and the *conditioned response*. He showed that a *conditioned response* occurs when an initially neutral stimulus becomes associated with an involuntary response by its association with a previously conditioned stimulus. He paired the introduction of food with the ringing of a bell, and found that eventually dogs would develop the reflex of salivating merely to the sound of the bell, even in the absence of food.

He also found that this *learned* conditioned response could be *unlearned* by reversal of the stimulus, *magnified* by repetition of the stimulus, or *extinguished* over time by the withdrawal of the stimulus.

Classical conditioning of fear almost certainly occurs in dental patients who undergo repeated painful procedures, and can also occur where minor pain and intense emotional arousal have been paired. It can also form associations between the environment surrounding a painful event and emotional processing of that event, so that the environment alone could trigger the emotional dimension of pain. Fear-conditioning may thus contribute to phobic behaviour in dental patients.

John Watson and Rosalie Rayner[18] illustrated that Pavlovian conditioning applied to human learning as well as to animals. Their experimental subject, the eleven-month-old (and very unfortunate) "little Albert", was known to be frightened by loud noises. Watson and Rayner conditioned him to fear a white rat by striking an iron bar with a hammer while repeatedly presenting little Albert with the white rat. Although initially Albert had no fear of the rat, he quickly developed a fear response through its association with the noise.

A further observation was that of stimulus generalisation. Little Albert then began to exhibit fear in the presence of similar stimuli such as a rabbit, a dog and a fur coat. Watson and Rayner were thus able to hypothesise that apparently irrational fears may be based upon the generalisation of a conditioned response.

In the context of dentistry an initial neutral response to a dental surgery can become associated with a stimulus such as a painful episode or a dentist perceived as cold or judgemental, giving rise to a conditioned response of generalised fear relating to dentistry. Repetition of these stimuli may lead eventually to dental phobia. Stimulus generalisation is shown by a person who, having experienced an unpleasant episode in a hospital, may develop a conditioned response of fear relating to a white coat, injections or a particular antiseptic smell. This response may then be activated when they attend a dental surgery.

The aim of treatment in such cases may be to pair a pleasant experience (e.g. relaxation and comfortable imagery) with the conditioned fear response, so that the phobia is extinguished. This is known as *systematic desensitisation* or *graded exposure*. The enhanced qualities of relaxation, visualisation and affect accessible through hypnosis make it an ideal agent for carrying out a desensitisation programme.

Operant conditioning

B. F. Skinner[19] succeeded Watson in the further advance of the behaviouristic approach to psychology. An early observation made by Skinner was that behaviour is likely to be repeated if followed by reinforcement. Through experimentation with laboratory animals he demonstrated that reward-based behaviours become reinforced by repetition, and may become extinguished rapidly in the absence of reinforcers.

Skinner's approach to the emotional behaviour that accompanies a deep fear or phobia is to suggest that this response is learned, for example as a result of the punishing consequences of some past behaviour in a particular previous situation. In the dental setting a patient whose previous dental experience was "punished" by pain or by a disapproving or apparently non-sympathetic dentist can readily develop an aversive behaviour that demonstrates itself by non-attendance and/or deep fear.

A dental patient who receives "applause" following a successful dental treatment session will be more likely to repeat and improve their behaviour pattern. This philosophy is a basis of *ego-strengthening* (Chapter 7), a powerful reinforcing process that should accompany almost all hypnotic interventions. Following a successful visit to the dentist and hypnotic ego-strengthening, a patient is likely to feel more comfortable about making another appointment. However, where there is "punishment', for example pain, or a dentist who is perceived as cold and unfriendly, there may be increased anxiety at future visits.

Cognitive theories of anxiety

These propose that cognition and information processing have a central role in anxiety. Anxiety and fear are conceptualised as adaptive mechanisms activated when there is the possibility of danger[20]. Whether fear or anxiety results from a given threat depends on a person's interpretation of the situation, which takes place in two phases. The primary appraisal – is that person's "domain" affected and is the threat imminent and likely to involve physical or psychological injury? – is followed by the secondary appraisal – what resources does the person have to cope with the threat? Anxiety can be seen as the result of an imbalance between the threat and the person's ability to cope[2, 20].

The process may be distorted in anxiety disorders by the person's misinterpretation of physical symptoms of anxiety (for example, in a panic attack) or by an exaggerated sense of vulnerability so that the person focuses on their weaknesses rather than their strengths. Negative thoughts and expectations of things going wrong are characteristic of anxious dental patients, and even when they have a successful (i.e. pain-free and not distressing) dental visit, they may modify their memories over time to remember much more pain and distress than they reported at the time[21].

Hypnosis can be used to increase the perception of being able to cope, teach new coping skills and affect the memory for bad experiences, so that cognitive strategies can be improved.

Observational learning

Albert Bandura[22] proposed that voluntary and involuntary behaviour patterns may be learned by observing a significant other person's behaviour. The significant others on whom most children will model their behaviour will be parents or siblings. It is important to note that such modelling can have positive or negative outcomes. For example, behind many frightened children there is a similarly dentally anxious parent.

Modelling has been shown to be effective in reducing anxiety, particularly in children. It is important that the child sees the model not only undergoing the treatment but also showing cooperation and receiving praise for their good behaviour. It may also be important that the model is close in age to and of the same sex as the patient[23].

Hypnosis is characterised by heightened suggestibility and an enhanced ability to fantasise. This makes it a potent adjunct to the modelling process. In treating a person who is frightened by an aspect of dentistry, we can suggest a metaphor such as "... I was treating someone [*described subtly to match to the patient*] a few months ago who was really scared, but by the end of treatment he just told me how easy it had all been ... and how proud he felt when he looked in the mirror and saw his teeth looking so good ...".

In hypnosis children enjoy fantasies involving heroes film, TV or sport. These figures can be portrayed as ideal role models in the dental situation (see George, page 247).

Memory and pain perception

The emotions associated with an event will influence the memory of that event, and memories of past experience tend to shape expectations for the present and future[24]. In dentistry this can create distortions in which the recalled pain intensity is exaggerated within the memory. Because hypnosis has effects on memory we can use it to modulate the patient's recall of a dental treatment session, thus breaking the vicious circle of memory modification that keeps anxiety high.

Cognition, assumptions and pain perception

The stimulus–response sequence is governed by our appraisal of an occurrence, and this appraisal is influenced by past experience and present significance[2]. The patient will be making a number of *assumptions* about their pain based upon the question "how does that stimulus fit into my map of the world?" Factors influencing this will include history, previous experience, fears of outcome, current psychological/emotional/physical state and the stories of others.

Almost inevitably feedback from the negative emotions will increase the intensity of the response, thus setting up an ascending spiral of physical and emotional discomfort. For many people the only way of avoiding this situation is by avoidance behaviour, in other words non-attendance at the dentist.

As a result, the assumption of such a patient may become that dentistry is inevitably associated with pain and unbearable feelings and emotions, creating problems for both dentist and patient, and serving to amplify even further that person's negative response.

Overview

Dental patients contend with the negative emotion associated not only with pain's presence but also with its anticipation and its aftermath. Therefore the suffering of a patient is less a direct consequence of the sensory intensity of that patient's pain than of the distress the pain causes. Often the emotional component of pain depends heavily on the duration of the pain and the individual's view of themselves as being strong enough to tolerate it.

The Management of Fear and Anxiety

Panic feelings

Explaining to the patient

It is important that you put the panic into a more manageable context for the patient. First, gently encourage them to give a detailed background to their problem, and follow this up with a simple explanation of their symptoms, obviously tailored to that person's intellectual capacity. This will give them an insight into what is going on, and show them that you are familiar with the problem. It also reassures them that phobia and panic are not rare or a sign of madness or a cause for shame, and will begin to show the patient that the phobia is controllable.

The next part of this cognitive readjustment is to explain to the patient that the physical feelings that they are experiencing are not in themselves a threat, but are identical to the physical feeling of "love at first sight" or the anticipation of something exciting. Emphasise that is the *interpretation* of these feelings that converts them into the panic attack.

As an example, a description used by one of the authors goes something like this:

> "... this probably sounds a bit odd, but do you know Elvis Presley's song 'All Shook Up'? In the song he sings ... 'my hands are shaking and my knees are weak ... I can't seem to stand on my own two feet ... my inside shakes like a leaf on a tree' ... and he then says that it's great because it means he is in love! ... but the feelings are exactly the same as yours. So maybe we can start to help you to see these feelings in a different light ... what do you think?"

Having had this view understood and affirmed, you can suggest that through hypnosis the patient can learn to put a new perspective on the feelings of a panic attack, and through that learn to control their fear and cope with dentistry.

Breathing away the fear

This is a useful form of induction coupled with a method by which the patient might learn a sense of control and distraction from their anxiety. When the patient is seated, ask them to close their eyes and relax as far as they feel they can, and suggest the following:

> *"... I wonder if it's possible to blow a little of that anxiety away ... blow it away with each breath that you breathe out ... really slowly ... really gently ... I wonder if you can imagine that the anxiety has a colour ... what colour do you think it is? ... and each time you breathe out ... gently ... it's as though you're blowing out a cloud of colour ... as though you're gently blowing away that fear in coloured clouds ... aware of the warmth of the breath as you breathe out that coloured cloud ... and the slightly cooler, calmer, easier breath ... as you breathe in that calming air ..."*

As the patient gets into the breathing rhythm, you may then pace your suggestions in such a way as to slow down their breathing, gently leading this into any preferred deepening mode.

Anchoring

Because of the nature of dentistry and the relative position of patient and dentist, a hand on the patient's shoulder is a natural form of reassurance whether or not you are using hypnosis. However, when you have shown the patient the effectiveness of this form of anchoring in hypnosis, it can become particularly effective in giving the patient a sense of stability and security when it appears that self-control may be slipping during a clinical procedure

Nevertheless, there are some patients for whom this form of physical contact is not comfortable and you should always use your discretion when considering this approach.

When once the anchor has been accepted and learned it is quite natural and very effective to use it whether or not the patient is in hypnosis.

Desensitisation (after Joseph Wolpe)

Joseph Wolpe[25] was born in South Africa and studied at the University of Witwatersrand in Johannesburg. Dissatisfaction with psychoanalysis led him into the study of behaviour, which in the early 1950s led him to develop therapies aimed at easing a person's mental distress by altering their behaviour.

He found that if a person can be taught to replace his normal anxiety response to a stimulus by a response (say) of calmness and tranquillity, then the fear and anxiety relating to the stimulus will become extinguished, because it is impossible to be relaxed and anxious at the same time.

Although Wolpe was known to have used hypnosis, generally relaxation was induced by progressive relaxation based on the work of Edmund Jacobson, and could be extremely time-consuming, sometimes taking up to 200 sessions[26]. Wolpe's own figures show that for "simple neuroses" the average number of therapeutic sessions required was fifteen[25]. Hypnosis is therefore a remarkable facilitator, as for many patients a profound state of relaxation may be produced within a few minutes, thus speeding up the entire therapeutic programme. Wolpe's technique became known as "systematic desensitisation by reciprocal inhibition".

We can apply this principle in the management of a dental patient's fear and anxiety. In this context the aim is to teach the patient, within hypnosis, to replace their fear response with one more appropriate, usually incorporating emotions of calmness, control and success.

Hypnosis is a of particular value in formal desensitisation for a number of reasons:

Rationale for hypnosis in desensitisation

a) As phobic individuals have been shown to be on average more highly hypnotisable than the rest of the population, hypnosis suggests itself as the treatment of choice[27].
b) Hypnosis facilitates profound relaxation easily and quickly.
c) It enhances fantasy, visualisation and affect.
d) It reduces the degree of emotional inhibition.
e) It is easily controlled by both the dentist and the patient.
f) It is easy to move from "in vitro" to "in vivo".
g) Hypnosis helps to build rapport, thus maximising the placebo effect.

Desensitisation programme in dental practice

1. The first step is for the patient, either alone or with prompting, to produce a "hierarchy" – a written list of anxiety-provoking situations beginning with the least severe and continuing through to the most fearful. For example, such a list may cite at Number 1 "receiving my appointment card" and progress through to Number 10, "having an extraction".
2. Take the patient into hypnotic relaxation, and encourage them to recognise how good this state feels.
3. Set up an ideomotor signal response. This stage is particularly important.
4. Encourage the patient to enter a hypnotic "good place", with the accent being placed on calm, controlled success. Ideomotor signalling will indicate when they have attained this.
5. Set up an anchor (for example, hand clench or finger-thumb), relating to this particular place and the feelings evinced.
6. Ask the patient to signal that they are prepared to fantasise the first item of their hierarchy, and if so encourage them to do so with your input. Then encourage them

to take this experience to an emotional peak before engaging the anchor to collapse that negative feeling and replace it with the original calm positive feeling. At this stage encourage them to note their success and how pleasant the relaxation feels.

7. You may then ask the patient to indicate whether they wish to move higher up their hierarchy. The style of questioning is critical as the patient can only indicate "yes" or "no" and the options may be:
    "Do you want to repeat that stage?"
    "Do you want to move to the next stage?"
    "Do you want to move several stages on?"
    "Do you want to stop?"

8. Repeat the process according to the patient's expressed needs.

9. At each stage introduce ego-strengthening based on the patient's performance.

10. Then alert the patient and invite them to start experiencing dentistry *in vivo*, knowing that their anchor can be used during any procedure, and that you will be prepared to stop at any time if the patient so desires.

Ego-strengthening and post-hypnotic suggestions

It should become a routine to incorporate ego-strengthening post-hypnotic suggestions just prior to alerting the patient from any procedure, and particularly when using such techniques as anchoring and desensitisation.

> *"... you'll be really pleased when you remember how you feel right now ... how well you've done ... how good it feels ... how you've overcome those fears and actually got your teeth fixed so easily ... each time you use self-hypnosis you'll find it becomes easier, that it works more and more effectively, more quickly, more deeply ... with a greater and greater effect over the way you think ... and feel ... and behave ... and you'll feel excited and pleased with yourself about this programme ... and about the things you've achieved today ... and as a result you'll feel comfortable and relaxed prior to your next appointment ... and when you come and sit in the dental chair next time you'll feel so very relaxed ... at the appointment, happy to sit in this chair, and when appropriate go into deep relaxation ... much deeper even than now ..."*

The above techniques might be used in conjunction with fear and pain management methods as described in the next part of the book. As dental anxiety is by far the most common condition you will treating with hypnosis, many of the chapters of this book will contain alternative techniques.

25

The Management of Pain

Our aims in using hypnosis within pain management are threefold:
1) To reduce or eliminate pain during a dental procedure.
2) To do this without otherwise affecting that patient's behaviour.
3) To teach the patient self-hypnosis in order that they may become self-reliant, self-confident and autonomous regarding future dental treatment.

Hypnosis is a quick, effective and safe method for raising the pain threshold and increasing pain tolerance. Through hypnosis the patient can be taught to address the physiological, cognitive and emotional expressions of the pain experience, enabling the alleviation of the pain itself together with reduction of suffering, distress and anxiety evoked by it. By these means we can enable the patient to develop an increased sense of mastery, independence and self-control.

In hypnosis we can directly suggest alterations in pain perception. Hypnosis can also be used to produce profound analgesia, sometimes sufficient for surgical intervention without chemical anaesthetic agents, although in practice we would generally use hypnosis in conjunction with conventional local anaesthesia.

Strategies in pain management

General rules
Although hypnosis can be a highly effective tool in pain management, certain key elements should always be borne in mind.

In procedures with the potential to cause pain, simply suggesting that "there will be no pain" is a negative suggestion and should be avoided. If you suggest that "you won't feel anything" the patient will not believe you, and in any case he will inevitably feel something. It is far better to explain what he will feel, not what he won't feel. It is sensible, therefore, to give the patient an explanation of what is about to happen, and why it is about to happen.

You may also be faced with a patient who presents in such pain that you need to reduce it before definitive treatment can begin. Simple techniques can be used quickly and effectively:

> *"... pain almost always makes us feel tense ... and then that tension seems to make the pain worse ... so I'm going to show you how you can break out of that loop ... and as you become less tense ... more relaxed ... so you start to feel more comfortable ... more easy both in your mind and in your body ...*
>
> *... and as that happens ... so your pain gently starts to get easier ... starts to lessen ... until bit by bit you'll feel so relaxed that it will just flow away ... and you'll feel so good ..."*

Note that the sequence of events is sensible and self-explanatory and at the same time lets the patient see that by his own actions he can start to take control of this previously "uncontrollable" pain.

Suggestions that modify the character of the pain will often be much more effective than suggestions of complete removal of the pain, as the patient will often be able to relate them to the reality of what he is feeling. For example, a sharp pain may become "a tingling sensation", or the injection of local anaesthetic can be described as "... maybe you are aware of slight pressure".

Control

For many patients their fear of dentistry is based upon the feeling of being out of control, so it becomes essential when carrying out any hypnotic procedure, and particularly any that incorporates analgesia, that you make the patient aware that ultimately they are in control. You must emphasise that if at any time the patient wants you to stop for any reason they can instantly let you know and you will immediately stop what you are doing.

This may involve the use of ideomotor signalling (Chapter 8) or agreeing a signal with the patient, which may be simply that they are told to raise their left hand if at any time they wish you to stop. And reassure the patient that you will instantly do so.

The words we use ... reframing

It is critical to remember that many words in everyday use in the surgery, for example forceps and excavators, may convey a huge threat to the hyper-suggestible nervous patient. Consequently, it is fundamental that all staff are trained to use acceptable euphemisms, and never to use words that might carry a negative connotation.

You can also maximise the placebo effect of the techniques and materials you are using by the way in which you describe them. For example, your topical local anaesthetic gel might become "... new, really strong ..." or "... a magic cream ...". Also maximise the positive outcome by reframing suggestions: "the water is washing away all the bad bits ...", "... think how good you are going to feel ... and look".

The meaning of the pain

Beecher[28] noted that soldiers wounded in battle reported less pain and needed less medication than civilians similarly injured in car accidents. He hypothesised that the *meaning* of pain – in this case the good outcome of discharge from battle – was influential in a person's perception of the severity of pain.

From this we can see the importance of emphasising the good outcome in dental treatment in terms of improved health, function, comfort and appearance as well as the huge ego boost of completing treatment successfully. If these suggestions are given while the patient is in hypnosis, the impact upon pain perception is potentiated.

Case history: Geoff – the meaning of the pain

Geoff Graham was a dental surgeon; a larger than life character who was hugely influential in the promotion and teaching of clinical hypnosis in the UK and worldwide. The operation upon him here described was recorded, and has been used for teaching purposes.

The patient

Geoff, a very self-confident man of 65, was accomplished at using self-hypno-analgesia for dental restoration work. One day he arrived at his dentist as an emergency when the root holding a post crown on an upper lateral had fractured, remaining embedded deeply in the gum. He was extremely concerned about his appearance and potential sepsis, and said that when the time came to have the root surgically removed he would use self-analgesia.

Treatment plan

The plan was to construct a small partial denture to be fitted as an immediate replacement at the same appointment as the removal of the root, and at a later stage to replace this with a fixed bridge. Impressions were taken straight away, and the denture processed and made ready for fitting a week later.

Procedure

When Geoff attended for the removal of the root, he made himself comfortable in the dental chair, said *"I'm just going off on holiday"*, closed his eyes, relaxed deeply, and about two minutes later a smile best described as "beatific" spread across his face and he said in a sleepy voice, *"Right, let's go."*

Removal of the root was quite difficult and entailed gum flap preparation, removal of alveolar bone and trans-septal elevation of the two fragments. During this 30-minute operation there were moments when Geoff's smile evaporated and an

---

apparent tension spread through his face and body. Each time this happened the surgeon paused and made reassuring noises, and Geoff took a deeper breath and resumed his deep relaxation with the smile on his face. On completion, two sutures were inserted and the partial upper denture fitted successfully, and after about 20 seconds he opened his eyes, looked in the mirror and was obviously highly delighted by the result.

Afterwards Geoff explained the episodes of tension thus to his dentist:

"Most of the time I was away on a sunny beach and virtually unaware of anything at all in my mouth. Just occasionally it was as though I was observing what you were doing and I became pretty tense and so I would change the thought process and would tell myself that I was getting rid of the poisons and the rubbish and it would look great when it was finished, and with that feeling of security I went back to the beach."

Summing up
This seems to be a good example of the proposal by Beecher that pain perception can be mediated by the prospect of a good outcome, and was a valuable learning experience for all who saw the video of the operation.

Non-hypnotic strategies

Refocusing concentration

Even without using hypnosis you can bring about pain and anxiety reduction by simple displacement of the patient's concentration and attention. It was said of US President Gerald Ford that he stumbled on a State occasion because "he found it difficult to walk and chew gum at the same time". Although the claim was meant to be ironic, it contains an element of truth in that we cannot give two simultaneous events our equal individual attention.

Patients often tend to hold their breath while undergoing unpleasant procedures. We know that it is almost impossible to tense up during exhalation, so by suggesting that the patient concentrates upon breathing out during an injection we are using a distraction technique that is also working at a physiological level.

"... now please take a deep breath and hold it ... and concentrate as hard as you can on letting that breath out ever so slowly [begin the injection] ... no ... even slower than that ... really slowly ... concentrate on letting the breath out so-o-o slowly ..."

Relaxation techniques

Simple relaxation can be an effective form of pain management, and hypnosis is an excellent medium for facilitating this. Anxiety and relaxation are incompatible. It is impossible to be anxious and relaxed at the same time, so the process of extinction of dental anxiety can be enhanced by the use of hypnotic relaxation techniques.

Although the impact of relaxation upon pain perception is largely psychological, an obvious advantage of muscular relaxation is that the injection of anaesthetic fluid meets less physical resistance because of the relaxed tonus of any muscle fibres involved.

Hypnotic strategies

Indirect suggestion (after Dave Elman)

In this technique note that the initial remarks establish a subtle "yes set"[29], following which simple induction and relaxation is followed by a by-pass of the *critical faculty*, the patient's normal appraisal, analysis and reality-checking of suggestions and situations.

> *"You know every time you come for treatment we both notice how tense you get, and when you sit there with all that tension it just makes you feel more and more discomfort at whatever I happen to be doing. If I could teach you how to relax, your visits to the dentist could be made so much easier, and I'm sure you know that.*
>
> *So how would you like to enjoy a dental visit for a change instead of being all tense about it? All right, I'm going to show you how to relax. Take a long deep breath. Great. Now watch my hand come down over your eyes and your face. And just close your eyes. And relax your eye muscles to the point where they won't work ... and when you are sure they won't work, test them to make sure they won't work. That's terrific. Now just stay like that and let that feeling of relaxation that you have in your eye muscles go right down at your toes.*
>
> *Now I'm going to lift your hand and drop it and if it's really as relaxed as it can be it'll drop down onto the armrest just like a wet tea towel. That's great. Now I'm going to go ahead with treatment to get your teeth into fantastic shape and nothing from now on will bother you or disturb you at all.*
>
> *You'll know that I'm working in your mouth. But as you hold on to that relaxation you will stay absolutely comfortable. You'll know that I am working but it won't bother you the slightest bit."*
>
> [Lead into direct suggestion.]
> *" and as we work you can let your mouth and tooth feel completely numb ..."*

Counting while injecting local anaesthetic

This is a simple and effective way of facilitating the injection of local anaesthetic. Although it is in itself a form of hypnotic induction, it may be helpful if you begin by carrying out your normal induction before seamlessly introducing the following:

> *"... as you lie there relaxed and calm ... just feel your body relaxing and letting go more and more with each outgoing breath ... aware that your muscles are so comfortable and relaxed ... and the muscles around your face are really relaxed ... so that you can just let your lips come apart as your mouth gently falls open ... effortlessly and easily ... and as it does so feel your body becoming even more comfortable and heavy in the chair ... and you can just allow yourself to focus on the sound of my voice ... just on my voice ... and I'm going to slowly count to ten ... and as I count to ten let your mind totally focus on each number ... focus so deeply on each number that I count ... totally concentrated on nothing but my voice and on each breath that you breathe out ... relaxed and calm ... one ... even deeper ... two ... deeper still ..."*

As you count, slowly and gently introduce the syringe into the patient's mouth and insert the needle slowly and smoothly in one steady movement. Equally slowly and smoothly begin injecting the local anaesthetic. If at this stage you note any slight resistance or tension, you might acknowledge this by congratulating the patient on their achievement so far, introducing ego-strengthening, and at the same time reframe the situation. For example:

> *"... you may be aware of a bit of pressure or a slight tingling feeling ... and that's absolutely normal ... and it shows that it's working properly ... so you can relax even more ...".*

If at any time the patient reacts more strongly or brings in their prearranged "stop" signal, it is important that you comply with this, acknowledge their problem and reintroduce hypnosis. You might then congratulate the patient on how well they have done as a means of ego-strengthening, and check out with them the immediate cause of the problem. With reassurance many patients will then be prepared to go through with the procedure.

The mental holiday

This method simply employs the use of imagery with the added suggestion that the patient may reinterpret and integrate into the hypnotic daydream any sensations, physical or auditory, that he may experience.

> *"... don't you think it would be great if you could somehow just take your mind off on holiday while you leave your teeth here for me to fix? ... OK, why don't we do that ... soon I'm going to help you find somewhere that you can just go off to ... it might be somewhere peaceful and relaxing ... but it might be just something you enjoy doing ... anything ... a hobby ... sport ... going on holiday ... anything ... and while you're there you might just be aware somewhere at the back of your mind that I'm working in your mouth ... or you might not ...*

> *but it will feel so good to be where you are that all of this will just fade into the background ... and you might be aware of certain sounds and certain sensations ... but they will just be in the background too and absolutely OK ... and you'll possibly even find that they become a part of your daydream ... help you to get even more deeply involved in it ... and you will probably become so involved in that daydream that time will go by really quickly ... and you know that if you were to want me to stop working you can signal as we arranged ... and I will instantly stop ... so now if you're ready maybe you could let that 'yes' finger let me know ... that's great ... let's make a start ..."*

Note that the imagery and visualisation here does not necessarily need to be calm and peaceful, the major criterion being that the patient can become so deeply involved in it that they spontaneously dissociate from the actuality of the dental work.

Time distortion

Time distortion is seen in our day-to-day life in that when we are enjoying something time "just seems to flash by" whereas when we are bored or suffering time "seems to drag". Many patients in simple relaxation and in hypnosis lose their consciousness of time. Patients when asked might report that a session has lasted about 15 minutes, when over twice that time might have elapsed. This phenomenon can be enhanced by direct suggestion[30].

> *"... while you're enjoying that beautiful dream you're enjoying it in hypnotic time, which is very different from real time, so that when I ask you to come back to full awakeness it may seem as if very little time has passed ... and all you'll remember of this experience is that it's been so pleasant and easy and enjoyable."*

Components of pain

Melzack and Wall[31] described three major components governing an individual's pain response to a stimulus:

1) **Sensory-discriminative.** This provides information about location and sensory quality of the stimulus (for example, "I've a sharp pain in my upper right central incisor").
2) **Motivational-affective.** This refers to the "bothersomeness" of the pain and may be mediated by a number of situational and emotional factors (for example, "I've got a blinding headache").
3) **Cognitive-evaluative.** This relates awareness of the *meaning* of the pain to that individual (for example, "this pain is unbearable").

So in dealing with pain management we are working with the combination of the physical sensation, the emotional suffering that goes with it and the person's evaluation of its meaning. Each system will influence the other two, so that the pain response is dynamic rather than static, and will be self-perpetuating, giving rise to a *feedback spiral*.

Separating the components

Joseph Barber[32] proposes a useful metaphor in helping a patient to distinguish between the *intensity* of pain and its affect, the *bothersomeness* of the pain. He suggests the analogy of listening to music, where on the one hand there is the volume or intensity of the sound that corresponds to the sensory component, and on the other there is the timbre and tone, the *bothersomeness*, which corresponds to the affective dimension of the pain.

This can be explained thus to the patient:

> *"Maybe you have noticed that when you hear a piece of music there are certain sounds that are so beautiful that you can listen and enjoy them even though it's really loud.*
> *But if there is discord or a harsh timbre or tone, even when you play it quietly it can be quite disturbing, and at a high volume it would be unbearable.*
> *So 'loudness' and 'bothersomeness' are not the same.*
> *Now I wonder if you could consider that pain you've had and rate it on a scale from zero to ten ... where zero is pain-free and ten is the most intense pain you could imagine.*
> *And similarly with the bothersomeness, where zero is when it doesn't bother you at all and ten is as bothersome as you can imagine.*
> *And even see that scale in your mind's eye.*
> [elaborate]
> *Now ... imagine that you actually have, just like on a sound system, a volume control and a tone control. And you can turn them to increase or decrease the volume and to make the sound sweeter and less harsh ... and as you relax more and more deeply, see yourself turning those two controls to levels right now so that it feels more comfortable for you ...".*

And this can all be incorporated into self-hypnosis, achieving three primary objectives:
a) It gives the patient a perception of *control* over the pain (a huge potential advantage in starting to manage it), and so the patient can learn to control the pain.
b) The balance that the patient describes can suggest to you, the therapist, entry points within the menu of techniques you may have in helping within pain management.
c) It gives an analogue scale for monitoring and evaluating progress during therapy.

Control centres

Control of the pain is a major issue for many sufferers. Through hypnotic imagery you can show the patient how to develop a sense of control, and feeding this control back into the spiral can result in dramatic pain reduction.

The patient can be taught to turn the pain down using a "control centre" in the brain, or by using dials or switches or a computer screen. Computer analogies may be useful – the patient might close down the pain programme, or debug the system to remove the pain virus.

The metaphor of thermostatic control will bring in other factors such as time lag and distraction:

> *"I wonder if you've ever been in a room when it's been too warm or too cold ... and you notice that on the wall is a thermostat to control the temperature in the room ... and next to it is a small dial that you can turn to adjust the temperature ... to turn it up or down in the direction that you want ... and it turns so easily ... and at first nothing seems to happen ... and then there's the slightest little click ... and it's so tiny that you hardly feel or hear it at all ... but you just know it's happened ... and although at first nothing seems to change in the room you know that somewhere that dial has connected with switches and machinery ... started to alter the settings on a huge boiler somewhere in the building ... and at first nothing in the room seems to have changed ... but then over the next few minutes and hours you become aware almost subconsciously that the room has cooled down or warmed up just as you wanted ... and so now, as you dream away, maybe you can see in your dream how within your mind ... right at the back of your mind ... there's a control you can turn ... and you can start to control how you feel ..."*

Almost all the descriptions that are used to describe pain take the form of metaphor ("shooting", "grinding", "burning"), and simile ("it feels like my head is in a vice"). It is vital that you take on board the precise metaphors or similes the patient uses, because these will give you the perfect pathway to hypnotic management of their pain. Furthermore, these descriptive words will tell you whether the patient's major preoccupation is with the sensory-discriminative or motivational-affective aspect of their pain.

Sensory components

You can give suggestions in hypnosis towards altering the way the patient thinks about their pain by modifying the imagery they have given you in their history. As the patient learns to do this and changes the experience of pain, they develop a sense of control over something they previously thought was uncontrollable.

It is important that you use your own imagination to *see* the images you are presented with (e.g. the tautness of a balloon, a hot knife, a tightly bound rope, a clamp or a vice) so that you can invent realistic strategies to modify them.

It is also important that you suggest realistic goals, a gradation of symptoms rather than immediate eradication (e.g. a "sharp stab" can become a "pressure with a blunt object" and lead into a "tingling sensation").

Table 25.1 **Modification of pain characteristics**

	Modification of pain characteristics
Feeling	Is the sensation sharp, stabbing, crushing?
Mobility	Does it move?
Colour	Does it have a colour? If so, what colour would signify comfort?
Physical	What is its shape, its texture, its appearance? Is it hard or soft? Is it light or heavy? (Maybe you can shrink, soften, smooth, mould, melt or dissolve it.)
Temperature	Is it hot? Or warm? Or cool? Or cold?
Displacement	Can you move it somewhere further away or more acceptable? (*"... you may sense the pain moving around in a spiral, going out further and further until it seems to have moved right down to your left hand, and seems much less bothersome ..."*)

Future pacing

Maybe it is possible to look towards a successful outcome. Through imagery the patient can be taught *forward pacing* in order to see themselves at some future time when they have learned to control the pain.

Direct diminution of sensation

"... you're starting to feel so good, and with each outgoing breath it's as though the discomfort is just gently flowing away ..."

Special place

In setting up "special place" imagery, utilise all the sensory modalities to create experience of really being there: "... completely relaxed and safe, imagining what you can see, hear and feel, even smell".

The feelings can then be enhanced by the creation of concepts such as magic healing pools and protective bubbles.

Glove analgesia

Glove analgesia involves teaching a patient in hypnosis to produce analgesia in a prescribed area of their hand which would correspond to a glove. When the patient has successfully demonstrated that they have done this they can be taught to transfer the numbness to an appropriate area, empowering them to produce dental self-analgesia.

Although most of the hypnotic techniques involved are conventional, there are certain provisos that are essential for the patient's understanding and cooperation and to guarantee their safety.

Explanation

It is vital that you describe to the patient what they are likely to experience in hypnotic analgesia, and answer any questions they may have about it. You might emphasise the fact that they will be in control of the analgesia and that you will not act without their consent, and you will stop work at any instant they may wish you to.

Explain that the state of analgesia will last for as long as they need it to, and that on reversing it they will feel absolutely normal – and extremely pleased with themselves.

Note that the altered sensation does not follow nerve distribution and will take place just where directed. Note also that unless a tooth is already hurting, the patient cannot tell whether or not it has gone numb. It is recommended therefore that the patient is encouraged to rub the relevant tooth together with adjacent mucosa and teeth, so that they can experience from the mucosa a sense of numbness.

Alerting

Following treatment and before the patient is alerted, a post-hypnotic suggestion can be given as follows:

> *"Your tooth and gum can remain numb and comfortable for as long as you need them to. When you and your body are ready, you can notice that the tooth and gum have regained their feeling."*

Language

As always, the language you use should be matched to the patient's own use of language and to their background and understanding of the situation.

If you are suggesting "it will feel like X", be certain that the patient knows what X feels like, and that what you are describing has a pleasurable connotation.

For example, do not suggest that "it will feel numb like a local anaesthetic", because the patient may not know what a dental injection feels like, hypno-analgesia does not feel like a dental injection, and for many patients a dental injection may have a very negative connotation.

Communication

Reassure the patient that they can maintain contact with you and will remain in charge of the situation. For this purpose a signalling system such as ideomotor signalling (Chapter 14) should be established. However, less formal signalling such as a nod or shake of the head (provided you are not working on a tooth at that time) or a simple raised left hand might be more than adequate.

As described in that chapter, in the dental setting it is normal to choose the left hand as the signalling hand as it is clearly visible in your sight line. For this reason it is normal in the dental situation to demonstrate hypno-analgesia on the patient's right hand.

Do not fall into the trap of numbing the signalling hand!

Time and situation bar

When hypno-analgesia is being used for the purpose of dental work it may be appropriate to give a certain time extension in order to cover any post-operative pain. Here you can either give the post-hypnotic suggestion that the numbness will last for another couple of hours before reversing, or ask the patient to use their own reversing procedure after the same time lag.

You should stress to the patient that on no account should any self-hypnotic analgesia be used in pain control where the reason for the pain is unclear or unknown. In fact patients should be warned only to use this technique in relation to pain where their doctor or dentist has specifically advised it.

Touching the patient

Inevitably there will be times when it is necessary for you touch the patient while they may have their eyes closed, for example when you are comparing the level of sensitivity in one hand against that in the other.

At all times it is essential that you caution the patient that you are about to do so, and this is described in an example script below.

Testing

In the examples given below it is suggested that analgesia is tested for by a gentle needle prick or needle insertion. A useful preliminary test that does not incorporate needles, and might be more suitable as a demonstration for the more nervous patient, is as follows:

> *"... I wonder if you've ever woken up after lying on your hand and found that your hand has gone to sleep ... just imagine that feeling ... feel it flow into your right hand ... so that the hand becomes numb and floppy ... just as if you've been lying on it and it's gone to sleep ... so that if I place this pen in your left hand you'll find you can grip it quite normally ...* [place a pen in patient's left hand and let them grip it as you try to remove it] *... but if I put it in your right hand ... the hand is so floppy and numb that it just doesn't grip it at all ..."* [demonstrate]

Limitations

Not all patients will achieve a deep, or even workable, level of hypno-analgesia, and the state is certainly not an "all or nothing" phenomenon. Whatever degree of success that patient achieves, be quick to congratulate them and to incorporate that success into further ego-strengthening.

Techniques for glove analgesia

There are numerous ways of inducing hypnotic glove analgesia and you might also like to bear in mind that any suggestions aimed at producing physical or perceptual change will also carry a strong deepening effect.

Glove analgesia by direct suggestion

> *"... as you relax more and more deeply ... you may become aware of a tingling feeling in the fingertips of your right hand ... and as you concentrate on the feelings and sensations in that hand ... you'll realise that gradually the tingling spreads ... just as far up as your wrist ... and gradually and slowly your hand starts to feel a bit different ... different from your other hand ... and it begins to go numb ... and as you relax even more ... that right hand is becoming quite numb ... more and more numb ... as if there's no feeling in your hand ... and soon I'm going to be counting to three ... and as I count that hand will become more and more insensitive ... so that when I reach three that right hand will be absolutely numb ... absolutely insensitive ... one ... more and more numb ... more and more relaxed ... two ... quite numb now ... deeper and deeper ... and three ... absolutely numb ... absolutely insensitive ..."*

At this stage, provided that the patient has indicated that their hand does indeed feel numb, you may want to give them (and yourself) a demonstration of the effectiveness of the analgesia:

> *"... now I'd like to show you how effective this numbness is ... and we can do that by comparing it with your other hand ... is that OK?* [get confirmation from the patient] ... *I'm going to touch your left hand with a pin and it might make you jump a bit ...* [the patient should react normally to a slight pin prick] ... *but now let's just see your right hand ..."*

Here you might push a hypodermic needle smoothly through a fold of skin on the back of the right hand and leave it in place, and generally there will be no reaction whatsoever from the patient, indicating the depth of analgesia.

> *"... in a moment I'm going to ask you to open your eyes ... but you will remain in this deep trance ... and you'll look at your right hand and see something that will both surprise and amuse you ... and then you'll close your eyes and go back into this deep state of relaxation ...*

Often the patient will smile and even laugh at the incongruity of the situation, and you can then remove the needle from their hand.

If there is no further therapy required at this time, all suggestions of altered sensation must now be reversed.

> *"... and now we can let your hand return to normal again ... and as it returns to normal maybe you can wriggle your fingers and realise that it's coming back to absolutely normal ... numbness and insensitivity completely gone ... and when that's happened open your eyes ... fully alert and back to here and now with me ..."*

Glove analgesia by stroking

An advantage of this method is that the physical contact involved will serve to increase rapport between the patient and yourself, it is perceived by the patient as a joint effort, and with a talented patient it can be carried out effectively in a very short time.

> *"... now I'm going to show you how you can get that right hand to go completely numb ... really quickly ... and what I'm going to do is to stroke that hand from the wrist down to the tips of your fingers three times ... OK? ... so please could you bend your elbow so that your hand is about 6 inches [15 cm] above the armrest ... thank you ..."*

Now take hold of the patient's wrist with your hand above and your thumb below and stroke slowly and firmly downwards right to the finger tips, slightly straightening out the fingertips each time. Each time, having reached the fingertips, simply reposition your hand at the wrist and pause for about 5 seconds before stroking downwards again.

> *"... so ... one ... I'm stroking down and as I do so your hand is starting to feel different ... maybe a little warm ... maybe a slight tingling feeling ... maybe even to start feeling a little numb already ... and you feel yourself relaxing even more deeply ... and ... two ... stroking down again ... deeper and deeper ... and now your hand can begin to feel quite numb ... right up to your wrist ... more and more numb ... more and more insensitive ... and ... three ... quite numb ... more and more relaxed ... quite numb now ... deeper and deeper ... absolutely numb ... absolutely insensitive ..."*

At which stage you may wish to continue as described above.

Glove analgesia with arm levitation

This can also be a highly effective and rapid method for the production of both deep relaxation and glove analgesia.

> *"... as you rest your right hand and arm on the armrest of the chair ... and you let yourself relax even more deeply ... you might become aware of one or two things that are starting to happen ... maybe a slight twitchy movement starting in your fingertips ... maybe a slight tingly feeling in your fingertips ... and as you relax even more ... and concentrate all your attention on that right hand you notice that your fingers start to rise a little ... rising away from the armrest ... as if they want to start floating upwards ... and as they do, so your hand is starting to feel different ... starting to feel numb ... starting to lose sensation ... as though your whole hand is feeling lighter and lighter ... and seems to want to float upwards more ... and ... as your arm gets lighter and floats upwards ... so your hand becomes more and more numb, until when I ask you to gently lower it you become so much more deeply relaxed ... and that hand becomes more and more numb ... until it becomes completely numb and insensitive ... so that by the time your arm and hand come to rest on the armrest ... you are so deeply relaxed ... and your hand is absolutely numb ..."*

Glove analgesia incorporating imagery

> *"I wonder if you can imagine that in front of you there is a deep bowl of water ... it may be a glass bowl or maybe it's ceramic ... it may be coloured or maybe not ... just signal to let me know when you can see it ... good ... and you realise that the water in the bowl is very, very cold ... maybe it's so cold that it's even got lumps of ice floating on the surface ... and when you can see that in your mind please signal to let me know ... thank you ... and let yourself become more and more deeply relaxed ... and now I wonder if you could put your right hand into the water ... just up to your wrist ... and you feel the cold ... really cold ... spreading through your hand ... and than gradually your hand starts to become numb ... more and more numb ... right through the skin and the muscle of your hand ... and when you can feel that feeling maybe you can signal to let me know ... that's great ... so that your hand is quite without feeling ... quite numb ... and when it's completely numb you take it out of the water ... and it remains absolutely numb ... totally insensitive ... all the way through ..."*

Glove analgesia incorporating a glove image

A gentle, effective and relatively passive technique for introducing glove analgesia is to suggest that the patient is wearing a glove that contains a powerful anaesthetic cream that pleasantly and gradually sends the hand numb. They can then remove the glove and retain the anaesthesia. You can elaborate on the imagery, and consequently the depth of involvement, by cueing the patient to look for detail in the image:

> *"I wonder what sort of glove ... maybe a mitten or maybe quite stylish ... leather ... or woollen? ... maybe you are aware of the colour of the glove ... the feel of it on your hand ..."*

Self-analgesia

When the patient has seen that they can produce hypnotic analgesia under your direction, it is comparatively simple for you to teach them how they can achieve this state for themselves on any appropriate future occasion.

First ask the patient to look down at their right hand and to concentrate hard on it. Suggest that they now stroke their own right hand with their left hand, from the wrist down to the fingertips, while slowly counting from one to ten. Advise them then that when they reach ten their right hand will be numb and insensitive, just as it was when you carried out the analgesic procedure with them.

The outcome of this exercise, in addition to its effectiveness in bringing about self-analgesia, is that it will serve as a self-hypnosis induction and consequently the creation of analgesia will tend to lodge in the patient's mind as a post-hypnotic suggestion.

Tell the patient that when their hand has become numb they should let you know, and then let both hands rest on the armrests. Both or either of you can then test their hand for analgesia as described earlier, and you can then ask them to alert themself from hypnosis in their usual manner, but to retain the analgesia in their hand.

It is important that you now demonstrate to the patient how they might bring the analgesia to an end and return their hand to normal. Invite them to choose a verbal signal such as "three, two, one, back to normal" or "the feeling's come back" that they can decide to use, and then get them to demonstrate this to you. The patient can then use this same signal for themself in order to restore normal sensation following self-analgesia.

Congratulate the patient on their (very real) achievement and re-impress upon them the precautions outlined above regarding limitations and safety precautions in its use.

Transferring the analgesia

The next stage is to empower the patient to transfer the numbness to their other hand, which has the double effect of showing that they are in control of the numbness and also preparing ultimately for transfer of the numbness to the tooth. First allow the patient, using self-analgesia, to produce numbness in their hand.

> *"... now the amazing thing about this numbness is that you can actually move it around ... what I'd like you to do is to place your numb left hand on top of your right hand ... and imagine that the numb feeling flows from the left hand into the right hand ... and in a moment, when that's happened, maybe you can let both your hands rest as they were before ... and if you'd now wriggle the fingers of your left hand to show me it's back to normal ... thank you ... and we'll just test your right hand with this pin and you'll find it's absolutely numb ...* [test it and let the patient see the testing] *... and so you can see that you can transfer that feeling wherever it's needed ... even to your teeth ..."*
>
> [At this stage it is appropriate to congratulate the patient, and important to caution them.]

> *"... so you can see that you have this fantastic ability ... and it can make dentistry so much easier and more comfortable for you ... and it is so important that you use this ability with care ... that you do not use it as a trick or to mask pain ... but only use it when here with me or another dentist to help fix your teeth ..."*

When the time has come to carry out dental work and the patient is in the dental chair you might say:

> *"... why don't you close your eyes and take yourself deeply into hypnosis as you normally do ... and ... when you are ready, bring up your hand and rub that tooth and all around that tooth until it's completely numb ... and when you've done that you can just drop your hand down again ... and when you're ready for me to start maybe you can just let your 'yes' finger twitch upwards so that I know ... and if at any time you want me to stop, just let your 'no' finger twitch and I will stop instantly ... and when I'm working you'll probably be aware of different noises ... like this for instance ...* [run the drill well away from the patient for a few seconds] *... and various sensations ... but as you just dream away you can let these fade into the background ... and they might even become part of this really pleasant dream ... and you can let your jaw muscles be so relaxed that your mouth just drops open ... OK, let's make a start ..."*

While you are working there is little necessity to speak apart from making gentle affirmative noises or warning the patient in a general way if you are going to be carrying out a more complex procedure or, for example, taking an impression.

At the conclusion of treatment carry out normal ego-strengthening, suggest that the patient lets all the feelings in their mouth and body return gradually to normal and, when they are ready, simply counts themself out of the hypnotic state back to full alertness.

References and suggested further reading

1. Rogers C. On Becoming a Person. London: Constable and Company Ltd, 1961.
2. Beck AT. Cognitive Therapy and the Emotional Disorders. Boston, MA: Meridian, 1976.
3. Heap M, Aravind KK. Hartland's Medical and Dental Hypnosis. London: Churchill Livingstone, 2002.
4. Wolberg LR. Hypnoanalysis. London: Heinemann, 1946.
5. Watkins J. The affect bridge: a hypnoanalytic and counterconditioning technique. Int J Clin Exp Hyp 1971;19:21–7.
6. Rossi EL. The Psychobiology of Mind-Body Healing. New York: Norton, 1986.
7. Wardle J. Fear of dentistry. Brit J Med Psychol 1982;55:119–26.
8. Forrest WR. Stresses and self-destructive behaviors of dentists. Dent Clin N Am 1978;22(3):361–71.

9. Hart BB. Hypnosis and pain. In: Heap M, Dryden W, eds. Hypnotherapy: a Handbook: Open University Press, 1991.

10. Hakeberg M, Berggren U, Carlsson SG. Prevalence of dental anxiety in an adult population in a major urban area in Sweden. Community Dent Oral 1992;20(2):97–101.

11. Skaret E, Raadal M, Berg E, Kvale G. Dental anxiety among 18-year-olds in Norway. Prevalence and related factors. Eur J Oral Sci 1998;106(4):835–43.

12. Chanpong B, Haas DA, Locker D. Need and demand for sedation or general anesthesia in dentistry: a national survey of the Canadian population. Anesthesia Progress 2005;52(1):3–11.

13. Nuttall NM, Bradnock G, White D, Morris J, Nunn J. Dental attendance in 1998 and implications for the future. Brit Dent J 2001;190(4):177–82.

14. Orwell G. Nineteen Eighty-Four. London: Essential Penguin Books, 1949.

15. Lautch H. Dental phobia. Brit J Psychiat 1971;119(549):151–8.

16. Locker D, Shapiro D, Liddell A. Negative dental experiences and their relationship to dental anxiety. Community Dent Hlth 1996;13(2):86–92.

17. Pavlov IP. Conditioned Reflexes. London: Oxford University Press, 1927.

18. Watson JB, Rayner R. Conditioned emotional reactions. J Exp Psychol 1920;3:1–14.

19. Skinner BF. Science in Human Behaviour. New York: Macmillan, 1953.

20. Beck AT, Emery G. Anxiety Disorders and Phobias: A Cognitive Perspective. New York: Basic Books, 1985.

21. Kent G. Memory of dental pain. Pain 1985;21:187–94.

22. Bandura A. Social Foundations of Thought and Action: A Social Cognitive Theory. Englewood Cliffs, NJ: Prentice Hall, 1986.

23. Kent G, Blinkhorn AS. The Psychology of Dental Care. Oxford: Wright, 1991.

24. Kent G. Memory of dental experiences as related to naturally occurring changes in state anxiety. Cognition Emotion 1989;3(1):45–53.

25. Wolpe J. Psychotherapy by Reciprocal Inhibition. Stanford, CA: Stanford University Press, 1958.

26. Jacobson E. Progressive Relaxation. Chicago: University of Chicago Press, 1938.

27. Gerschman, JA. Hypnotizability and dental phobic disorders. [Review] [38 refs]. Anes Prog 1989;36(4–5):131–7.

28. Beecher H. Pain in men wounded in battle. Ann Surg 1946;123:96–105.

29. Erickson M, Rossi E, Rossi S. Hypnotic Realities: The Induction of Clinical Hypnosis and Forms of Indirect Suggestions. New York: Irvington, 1976.

30. Hart BB. Hypnosis and Pain. In: Heap M, Dryden W, eds. Hypnotherapy: A Handbook: Open University Press, 1991, pp. 87–109.

31. Melzack R, Wall PD. Pain mechanisms: a new theory. Science 1965;50:971–9.

32. Barber J. Hypnosis and Suggestion in the Treatment of Pain. NY and London: Norton, 1996.

Habit Management

Habits are learned behaviours that have become automatic. Many habits are in fact beneficial; tooth-brushing is a habit that we wish all our patients could develop! Unfortunately, some habits are irrational and undesirable:

"Whenever I have a pint I just have to have a cigarette."
"When I am sitting reading or watching television I just start biting my nails."

Most habitual behaviours have served a real purpose at some time but have outlived their usefulness. Peer pressure is widely cited as the reason people start to smoke. Other habits may have been associated with feeling better in some way: the relief of tension by biting fingernails while watching a football match, relieving the stresses of the day by grinding the teeth together at night, or thumb sucking and smoking as a means of comfort. This has been termed the "positive intention" of the habit.

Smoking represents a special case because of the addictive properties of cigarette smoke. However, smokers will exaggerate the beneficial effects of tobacco. Some claim it is calming, stress-relieving and relaxing, and others that it stimulates them and makes them more alert. Indeed, if tobacco were capable of doing a fraction of what people claim it does, it would be the most versatile and useful drug known to man. The body instinctively knows when something is harmful. A "novice" smoker has to work very hard to become an "expert" smoker. The first-ever cigarette never tastes good and may even make the smoker feel nauseous. If that person believes he has strong reasons to be a smoker, he will persevere to establish the addiction. Once addicted the majority become enslaved, finding it impossible to escape no matter how hard they try.

Most smokers appear to be aware of the hazards; each year over 70% report wanting to give up smoking, with approximately 50% attempting to do so. Unfortunately, only 3–7% actually succeed without help[1]. Thus there is a real demand for professional help with smoking cessation.

Figure 26.1 **Some effects of smoking**

Some effects of smoking

Smoking is the greatest single cause of preventable ill health and premature death in the UK. Tobacco is the only legally obtained consumer product, that if used as directed, is likely to cause death or serious illness. The associated health risks have been widely publicised and include Cardio-vascular disease, Respiratory disease and Cancer. (For example, 80% of people who die of lung cancer are smokers.)

It is worth noting that;
traffic accidents kill approximately 5000 a year
heroin kills about 100 per year
smoking kills over 120,000 per year (13 people per hour)
(Ref: No Smoking Day Charity)

Diseases associated with smoking
Strokes
Defective vision
Aortic aneurysm
Heart disease
Vascular disease
Peptic ulcers
Gangrene
Respiratory disease
Cancer in most areas of the body

Diseases associated with passive smoking
Headaches
Asthma and allergies
Heart disease
10-30% more risk of Lung cancer
Cot deaths
Meningitis

Intra-oral consequences
Impaired wound-healing
Halitosis and bad taste
Staining and discolouration of the teeth
Over 90% of Oral cancer occurs in smokers
Periodontal disease

Many people find it difficult even to imagine life without the habit they have practised for so long, but hypnosis can be a powerful facilitator for change. The following chapters will outline hypnotic methods for the elimination of thumb-sucking, nail-biting, bruxism and, most importantly, cigarette-smoking.

General considerations for habit change

Dental personnel are unusual among health professionals in that we see patients regularly when they are not ill. Consequently we are in an ideal position to influence patients, particularly smokers, to modify maladaptive habits. Smoking behaviour should be noted as a routine part of history-taking and we should always give as much advice and support as the patient is willing to accept, including complimenting smokers who quit and encouraging those who have lapsed to try again to relinquish the habit. Leaflets and other information should be available.

Patients with maladaptive habits may be lacking in self-belief and self-esteem, so any treatment should include ego-strengthening, encouragement and development of the patient's self-confidence. The language used must be positive. Avoid phrases such as "I will *try* to" and "I *hope* I can" and especially "I *don't think* I can". As Henry Ford once said, "Whether you think you can, or think you can't, you're probably right."

Be supportive, sympathetic and non-judgemental when dealing with a patient's maladaptive habits. Emphasise that they *can* change and that they have the ability and the resources to change, rather than that they *must* change.

 Suggest that the patient approaches the change as a *challenge* rather than as a *problem*, and ideally develops a new behaviour pattern that is less harmful to them. Inform the patient that just as the original behaviour was ingrained with practice, so the new behaviour itself will in due course become automatic. At all stages stress the value of the new behaviour rather than the loss of the old behaviour.

Many of the habits we deal with are socially unacceptable in some way, be it the child embarrassed to start "big school" while still sucking their thumb, the nail biter embarrassed about their ugly hands or the smoker whose habit has recently been outlawed in public places and is increasingly frowned upon by the majority of the population. Therefore establishing rapport together with evident non-judgemental empathy is always an essential part of treatment. The patient must feel that you are on their side and it is essential that you do not appear condemning or condescending. Emphasising that you know how difficult it is to stop, and that you understand their situation, can be very reassuring. Some people may be ashamed or annoyed with themselves because they have failed to stop smoking (or nail biting etc.) either with treatment or without, and so it is important to stress right from the start that habits are difficult to break without help.

Motivation is extremely important and total commitment is required from the patient himself. Success is unlikely if the attempt to stop the habit is as a result of outside demands (or pressure from doctors and dentists).

Hypnotic strategies for habits

Some hypnotic strategies are appropriate for all habits. You should choose induction and deepening techniques that match the age and characteristics of the patient. Progressive muscular relaxation will always be useful and may form part of the core treatment when stress is involved in the maintenance of the habit. Ego-strengthening is essential and should always be included.

Teach self-hypnosis, with or without CDs or tapes, early on in the treatment sessions as this will increase the exposure of the patient to hypnotic techniques. The content of the self-hypnosis routine should be based on each individual's needs.

Occasionally habits are not just "empty" behaviours but are symptomatic of underlying problems, anxieties or other issues. If this is the case, then more psychodynamically orientated therapies such as regression or ego-state therapy may be indicated[2].

Reframing
Reframing is an extremely useful strategy in dealing with all habit disorders, its premise being that the habit has (or had) benefits for the person. Reframing helps the patient to adopt healthy behaviours, allowing them to discard the unwanted habit without feeling deprived of something that has served some purpose[3].

Six-step reframing

1) Contact the part responsible for the habit and acknowledge its excellent performance, but suggest that the positive intention can be separated from the behaviour.
2) Ask if the part is willing to become even more useful and effective.
3) Ask the creative part of the mind to generate alternative behaviour that allows fulfilment of the positive intention.
4) Ask the original part if it is willing to use any or all of those alternatives.
5) Have the patient carry out an "Ecology check" to ensure that no other part of their mind has any objections to the new behaviour.
6) The patient is asked to "Future Pace" – to vividly imagine all aspects of how their life will be without the unwanted habit.

Although formal induction is not essential, if used it can facilitate the processes involved and increase the patient's inner awareness and imaginative powers, allowing them to experience more vividly the life-enhancing effect of relinquishing the habit.

There does not appear to be a direct relationship between the "depth" of hypnosis and a successful outcome; often patients will achieve success without seeming to be greatly affected by the hypnotic procedure.

Many patients find reframing reassuring because it accepts that the habit was created to *help* them in some way. Instead of simply lecturing the patient on the unhealthy aspects, which would possibly alienate them, you are showing that you understand and respect the patient and their behaviour. Consequently there is much less chance of resistance from the patient, and they are more likely to feel that you are genuinely on their side.

Reframing also empowers the patient to do most of the work, encouraging them to use their own resources and thus enhancing their sense of self-belief.

Reframing in smoking cessation

1) Use the ideomotor response to communicate with the "smoking" part. Praise that part for doing exactly as it was asked to do, reassure the patient that there is no intention of getting rid of such a faithful part, and ask if it is willing to communicate. If the answer is "yes" –
2) Ask the part if it would consider becoming even more helpful by providing whatever it has been programmed to do, but in a way that is now more suitable. If the answer is "yes" –
3) Ask the creative part of the patient's mind to generate alternative ways for the original part to function, and to signal "yes" when this has been done. If the patient has difficulty here, suggestions can be given such as:
   • Taking deep breaths or breathing exercises
   • Chewing gum
   • Having a crystal, stone or other object that they can stroke or contemplate
   • Drinking some water
   • Doing something active such as walking or some other form of exercise.
4) Ask the part that "used to make you smoke" if it is willing to adopt this new behaviour. If the answer is "yes" –
5) Ensure that no other part has any objections to the proposed behaviour. If so, the "no" signal will be seen if there are no objections.
6) Finally, suggest that the patient imagines as vividly as possible what their life will be like without tobacco. Ask them to see, hear, feel, and even taste and smell how much better things are. Allow them as much time as they need to experience any situation or circumstance where they used to smoke, suggesting in a very positive way that they are very much aware of how much their lives have improved. Ask for a "yes" signal when they have spent enough time doing this.

It is most important to stress the positivity of being a *non-smoker* rather than the negativity of *stopping smoking*. The patient is not being deprived of anything. On the contrary, they are *gaining* better health, fitness and all the other benefits that prompted them to make the effort to stop. Likewise, you can suggest that when they are with other smokers, far from feeling envious of their smoking, they actually feel sorry for those people as they are still slaves to that addiction. The patient can be proud of their achievement in breaking free.

The session should always close with ego-strengthening suggestions, and a reminder to use self-hypnosis as previously directed. Suggestions can be given to help restrict the amount of weight gained. These may include advising sugar-free gum or sweets or drinking water, or other more specific dietary advice to suit that patient. Major elements of the session can briefly be reviewed and reinforced before alerting the patient. After making sure the patient has no queries or problems with the therapy, and after congratulating them, the patient can leave with instructions to be in contact after a week or so "to let me know how well you are doing". You may prefer to contact the patient yourself for this follow-up, as not all patients will make further contact.

27

Bruxism

Effects

The effects of bruxism can include muscle pain, TMJ problems and tooth substance loss, leading to sensitivity and pathology of the pulp. Diagnosis is made on the basis of symptom reports, including reports of noises disturbing sleeping partners. Bruxism may be nocturnal or waking, and may be present in both adults and children.

Aetiology

The aetiology of bruxism is uncertain but may involve abnormal occlusion, degenerative joint disease, congenital abnormalities, neoplasm and trauma. Before contemplating the use of hypnosis, it is essential to ensure that any organic cause is diagnosed and treated specifically.

However, as bruxism may be an expression of tension or anxiety[4, 5], hypnosis should be extremely effective in treating it. Unfortunately, evidence in the literature so far is confined to case reports[6-8] and a pilot study[9].

It has been suggested that the behaviour is an attempt to express any pent-up emotion, especially anger and frustration, and is a physical outlet as the brain processes whatever has occurred during the day.

Treatment options

Relaxation

Using hypnosis to increase the patient's ability to relax and deal with any anxiety is always helpful. Progressive muscular relaxation with emphasis on the muscles of mastication and other muscles of the head and neck can bring great relief. Suggestions to leave the teeth slightly apart, perhaps with the tongue just resting on the occlusal surfaces, can be incorporated into the relaxation programme.

Metaphors
Often patients respond very well to metaphors such as a rope or a rubber band slowly uncoiling and easing their tension. The metaphor should, as always, be matched to the background of the patient.

A chef, for example, may relate well to the image of spaghetti gradually softening, whereas a musician may find the idea of a guitar string loosening as the tuning key is turned more effective.

Glove anaesthesia
The technique can be employed to relieve any pain that has occurred in the muscles and around the TMJs or as a demonstration of control (see later).

Arm catalepsy
Arm catalepsy can be used to demonstrate to the patient that they have the ability to influence their muscular tension, and therefore if they can induce this rigidity in the muscles of their arm and then remove the tension, they have the ability to exert the same control over the muscles of mastication.

Post-hypnotic suggestions and self-hypnosis
Post-hypnotic suggestions can be used to "recondition" the habit.

> *"Each night you may say to yourself 'nothing is important enough to make me eat myself up'. One part of my mind will be instantly aware if my teeth touch, and this will make me smile as I acknowledge that my mind is trying to protect me.*
>
> *This will be the signal for me to relax and drift deeply into a wonderful, restful sleep".*

You can instruct the patient to use self-hypnosis each night to totally relax their jaws, and to allow this relaxation to persist throughout the night.

Anchoring
An anchor may be constructed with the suggestion that the jaw muscles will relax whenever the trigger is applied. This might be a word or a physical act such as pressing a finger and thumb together. Ask the patient to practise this before going to sleep to establish the link, and inform them that at the first sign of the unwanted behaviour starting the anchor will work, thus bringing the desired relaxation.

Ericksonian suggestions[10]

Suggest that the tension is transferred to another area of the patient's body, and that instead of the jaw muscles clenching it would be far more useful, and less damaging, for the hands to clench.

Erickson also suggested that the patient would awaken instantly if the teeth began to grind, and then the patient should get up and perform some tedious job such as cleaning the floors, the aim being that they would find it preferable to give up the habit rather than have their sleep disrupted.

Gow's hypnotic procedure for the treatment of nocturnal bruxism

An intervention has been developed that combines some approaches used previously together with some novel elements. This has been evaluated by the use of the Bitestrip® EMG unit, and was shown to reduce masseter activity and improve the habit in the opinion of the participants[11].

The intervention consisted of five visits (including the assessment visit). At the second visit induction and deepening and special place imagery were followed by relaxation strategies anchored by touching finger and thumb followed by a mantra of "Calm, control, and confident".

Ego-strengthening[12] was given and included the suggestions: "nothing is worth eating yourself-up over", and "your body is your most prized possession, take care of it". A further suggestion for automatic waking on grinding the teeth followed.

Visits 3 and 4 were tailored for each subject, taking the parts of the first session that they responded to best. In addition, glove anaesthesia (Chapter 25) was taught with the suggestion that if they could control sensation they could also control the bruxism habit. Patients were also taught self-hypnosis and given an audio-tape. This may be an important factor, as results showed a correlation between outcome and the use of these strategies.

Although this is a small study, it is the first to measure objective signs of bruxism (masseter activity) and to show positive effects of hypnosis when compared to a no-treatment control group.

Conclusions

Bruxism is a difficult habit to treat, and all traditional existing methods are under evaluation[13, 14]. Hypnosis adds another treatment option that may be successful.

Case history: Robert – bruxism and TMJ pain

The patient
Robert was a 40-year-old man with a very worn dentition who had developed severe pain in and around his right temporo-mandibular joint. He had previously been treated at the Dental Institute and had a soft appliance, which was not really helping at this time.

Hypnosis had been mentioned previously, and Robert declared himself ready to use hypnosis to alleviate this situation.

Treatment plan
To use hypnotic relaxation together with imagery appropriate to allowing Robert to become less tense and to sleep more easily.

Procedure
The first session involved taking a thorough history, which revealed that Robert was experiencing stressful events, especially at work.

Eye-fixation induction was followed by progressive relaxation, with specific emphasis on the muscles around his jaws. We had discussed some imagery before hypnosis and Robert had decided that imagining twisted sheets slowly becoming unwound and then smoothed out felt appropriate.

I also suggested that as soon as his teeth came into contact one part of his mind would be monitoring this and take it as a signal to relax and drift into a deep, untroubled sleep. An audio-tape was made of this session and Robert was asked to listen to this before going to bed each night.

At the end of this session, the pain seemed to be diminishing.

At the next visit, Robert reported that the severe pain had subsided, although he was still clenching and grinding his teeth.

Reframing and direct suggestions were used with ego-strengthening and a reminder to keep using the tape.

When Robert was re-hypnotised, an ideomotor response was set up, and I suggested that *"the part responsible for the grinding"* would respond to ideomotor suggestions. After acknowledging its good intentions, this part was asked to become even more helpful by altering the way it achieved its purpose by acting in a less destructive manner. This was agreed by ideomotor signalling. The imagery used previously was suggested again, with other direct suggestions that Robert would be more able to cope with any stressful events, and be much more aware of any tension anywhere in his body, especially his jaws, and therefore be able to release this tension. It was also suggested that *"... it will be interesting to see how quickly these changes occur ... with some people it is very quick ... whereas with others it takes a little more time ..."*.

I encouraged Robert to keep on using the tape for as long as he felt it was necessary.

Outcome

When I saw Robert two weeks later he was happy to report that he was sleeping better, the pain had gone and his teeth were not sensitive. He had made changes as far as his work was concerned and felt as though he was more able to cope with his life. According to his wife, he sometimes sighed or moaned on occasions, but she found that far less disturbing than the sounds of his teeth grinding together.

28

Gagging

The gag reflex is primarily a survival mechanism designed to prevent inhalation or ingestion of anything dangerous or unpleasant. However in many people this reflex becomes oversensitive, impeding necessary dental treatment or preventing oral hygiene from being carried out. We all gag if something touches far enough back in the mouth, so it is obviously very important to take the utmost care when taking impressions or radiographs or when working near the back of the mouth, and to be sympathetic and reassuring when doing so.

The severity of the reaction will vary from minor retches or choking when material or instruments touch the extreme posterior regions of the mouth to cases where the patient will start to gag at the very idea of a dental procedure. The intensity will also vary in that same person, depending on their health and mood at that time. People who find it hard to breathe through their nose may be more likely to gag.

Non-hypnotic strategies

Often the situation can be improved by taking time to explain, and letting the patient know that you understand and sympathise. Many people are embarrassed when they gag, feeling that they are being awkward and making it difficult for the dentist, or that there is something wrong with them. Carefully explaining to the patient that everyone has the reflex to protect them from injury and discomfort, and that they are not "mad or bad", can be most reassuring. You might add that in their case it's as though the mechanism is working *too well* and is being *over-protective*.

However, the gag reflex is not totally automatic. When we eat or drink the reflex normally stays dormant or we would not be able to ingest anything. This means that if a patient is able tolerate *some* substances touching these areas, it should be possible to extend this tolerance to other things. You might point out that people who do such things as swallow swords have practised increasing their control over this mechanism, and that compared to this, tolerating an impression or allowing a toothbrush near the lingual surfaces of the posterior teeth does not seem as impossible.

Often, taking the time to explain all this may be all that is necessary to allow the procedure to take place. You might ask the patient to imagine that the radiograph is a thin after-dinner mint, or that the impression material is something like porridge (ensuring that the food used as the example is not something that they find really unpleasant).

Giving simple suggestions of relaxation and calmness, especially with relation to their tongue, can help some patients manage, and there are various distraction techniques available, including the use of appropriate music. Some dentists ask patients to perform a variety of physical tasks, such as raising one leg or rotating one arm one way and the other arm in the opposite direction as a distraction during impression-taking. Some authorities advocate the use of a "sick stick". This is a wooden or metal rod about 45 cm (18 inches) long, which the patient holds. There is a mark in the middle of the stick and the patient is told that while they hold out that stick with both hands at arm's length and stare at the mark on that stick it will be impossible to gag. This distraction can overcome the gagging response for some patients.

Another technique that has an element of distraction employs acupressure.

The patient is asked to press one of their fingers on the midline between the lower lip and the point of their chin. This corresponds to the point known as Conception Vessel 24 (CV24). Sustaining pressure on this point can often allow dental procedures to be completed successfully, and can be used to increase the patient's tolerance to tooth-brushing and other oral hygiene procedures.

There will be some patients who will still be unable to overcome the gagging with the above methods, and more formal hypnosis can then be employed.

Hypnotic strategies

Anchoring
After hypnosis has been induced, anchoring to feelings of confidence, control and determination will enable the patient to feel more likely to succeed.

Emphasis on the potential advantages of successful treatment should be stressed. Benefits can include the improvement in appearance, speech and mastication that an edentulous person will achieve when they are able to tolerate dentures.

Through forward pacing the patient can be taught to imagine themselves having the required treatment successfully and tolerating the appliance or effectively maintaining their oral hygiene without gagging.

Finally, it is important to ensure that the patient will use self-hypnosis to continue rehearsing the anchoring process.

Desensitisation

A hierarchy can be established relating to the sensitivity of various parts of the mouth. The patient might decide that there is little or no reaction around the anterior teeth, but that gagging starts when anything touches the tongue, increasing towards the posterior teeth and even more so on the back part of the tongue, culminating in any contact with the soft palate initiating uncontrollable retching.

Through hypnotic imagery you can desensitise the patient to their hierarchy of fears in a step-by-step progression. When they have fantasised a successful outcome, it is important to expose them to the actual procedure as soon as possible. Quite often a radiograph or an impression can be taken immediately after hypnosis, without the patient gagging. With some patients it may be necessary gradually to extend their tolerance in reality.

In the treatment of denture intolerance the patient may be given a very thin acrylic plate, trimmed to the limit of their tolerance, and asked to wear the plate for longer and longer periods while carrying out self-hypnosis. The plate can then be extended at intervals until the patient can tolerate a functional denture. This graded desensitisation can also be used for impressions and radiographs, and can be potentiated and accelerated by the use of appropriate hypnotic relaxation and imagery.

Again it is important to ensure that the patient will use self-hypnosis to continue rehearsing their successful outcome.

Imagery

Ego-strengthening imagery should be used to increase the patient's sense of comfort, confidence and control.

As an example, you might invite the patient to imagine a small white cloud into which they place all the factors contributing to their problem. As this happens, they see the cloud grow darker and darker until it is full and there is nothing more to add. At that stage invite them to imagine the sun, and to see it shining and feel its warmth as it becomes brighter, burning away the cloud (and with it all the reasons for the problem). Suggest that as the cloud dissipates the patient gradually becomes more and more confident and capable of overcoming their problem.

Reframing

Through reframing the patient can be taught to modify their behaviour regarding gagging, so that they have sufficient tolerance to undergo the necessary treatment.

Dissociation

There are various techniques that make use of our ability consciously to detach ourselves from painful experiences, and many of these can be applied to the problems surrounding gagging. A useful phrase here is "Why don't you leave your mouth here with me and take your mind off on holiday?"

Split-screen techniques

Invite the patient to imagine a TV screen, a cinema screen or a theatre stage that is divided into two halves.

Suggest that they imagine that on one side is a very undesirable image for instance, their facial features sagging, their expression sad and ashamed, looking old and unattractive. They might also be asked to imagine themselves gagging.

Now suggest that the other side of the screen/stage contains a much more positive image. Here they see themselves smiling, feeling confident and in control, looking and feeling so good that they can undergo whatever is necessary to achieve and maintain a healthy, functioning mouth, with all the many benefits that this will bring.

Ask them then to concentrate on the side of the screen that they would prefer, and allow that side to become stronger, bigger and brighter, as the unwanted side gradually gets smaller and less distinct, eventually fading away until all that is left is the desirable outcome.

Where the emotional trauma is intense a form of *double dissociation* might be used. Here the patient is invited to imagine *seeing themselves* watching the scenes described above.

Regression

Occasionally, the problem will require a psychodynamic approach to uncover some underlying causes of the gagging, perhaps involving previous unpleasant experiences with impressions or other more disturbing events that gave rise to the present situation. Techniques such as affect bridge will often solve the problem, but sometimes this may require treatment from another therapist with the required expertise. As always, it is most important to know when a particular case is beyond your own area of expertise and be prepared to refer that patient appropriately.

Glove analgesia

You can teach the patient how to transfer the numbness generated by glove analgesia onto those areas that trigger the gagging, thus reducing the sensation to the extent that gagging no longer occurs.

Case history: John – Gagging

The patient
John was a 40-year-old man troubled by a strong gag reflex and a tongue that refused to let anything near the back of his mouth. He had always forced himself to attend regularly, even though he found dental treatment unpleasant and difficult. His oral hygiene, particularly posteriorly, was poor because of this problem.

Treatment plan
My plan was to use hypnosis in helping John to reduce his gag reflex in order to facilitate oral hygiene and necessary dental treatment.

Procedure

Following discussion about hypnosis, John realised its benefits and agreed to use it to improve his situation.

Induction was by an eye-roll technique coupled with counting down from the number 300. This was followed by progressive relaxation with emphasis on the muscles around John's jaws and tongue. Fractionation was used as a deepening procedure.

In hypnosis, I explained that everyone has a gag reflex and that it is a vital defence, preventing the swallowing or inhaling of harmful substances, but that in his case it was working too well and was too protective.

I explained that the good news was that his reflex was subjective and there were times when it was not triggered, usually when he had food in his mouth. I suggested that John could alter this mechanism to increase his tolerance, giving greater access for his toothbrush and for dental instruments.

I used sword swallowers as an example of people who had increased their tolerance enormously, stressing that the changes he needed to make were slight by comparison.

I reassured John that the basic reflex would be just as effective as a defence, there was no question of anything being removed or weakened, and that the reflex would simply become more flexible.

Self-hypnosis was taught, and John was encouraged to practise regularly, paying attention to relaxation, especially within his tongue. He was also asked to mentally rehearse the sensation of brushing his teeth and having dental instruments placed towards the back of his mouth, without the previous gagging or obstruction caused by his tongue.

A clenched fist physical anchor was set up to reinforce feelings of calm, confidence and control.

The changes have been gradual but definite, and treatment is far easier. John uses his anchor regularly and his oral hygiene is improving as his tolerance increases.

Access to the posterior areas has increased significantly and John is confident that he can continue to improve.

29

Thumb-sucking and Nail-biting

Both thumb-sucking and nail-biting involve placing digits in the mouth, thus introducing micro-organisms from digits into the oral cavity. Thumb-sucking can lead to varying degrees of malocclusion and sometimes deformity of the maxilla, whereas excessive nail-biting can cause loss of tooth substance resulting in sensitivity, as well as leaving unsightly hands and fingers.

Aetiology

Thumb-sucking is common in babies but becomes a problem when the habit persists after the child has started school. Nail-biting usually begins between the ages of six to twelve. Both habits can be a way of gaining attention, and often the behaviour is reinforced by parents constantly telling the child to stop doing it.

Both are conditioned responses that have become automatic, thus being outside of conscious awareness. Nail-biting will often accompany concentration or worry, or will take place while the person is watching TV or a football match. Thumb-sucking is a comfort to many people, possibly reminding them of suckling, and is generally a way of coping with anxiety, boredom or sleepiness.

Treatment options

Non-hypnotic treatments
Traditional treatments include aversion – usually painting substances that taste bad onto the fingers or thumbs[15] and a habit reversal technique including habit awareness, competing response training and social support[16]. Both have been shown to be successful[15, 17].

Hypnotic treatments

Most reports of hypnosis in treating these problems are confined to case reports[18-20]. Nail-biting has been studied in students and the study indicated that a hypnotic procedure improved success[21].

Direct suggestion

It is important to concentrate on the positive aspects of breaking the habit. For example emphasising the resultant improvements in appearance will motivate the patient to start making the change.

Direct suggestions can be given in hypnosis that the patient can change the bad habit towards better ways of behaving. Depth of hypnosis may be important in the success of this treatment[21].

Prescribing the habit

Methods of prescription aim to bring the habit into conscious awareness and may be direct or indirect.

Direct suggestion: "from this moment you will only be able to suck the thumb (or bite the nails) consciously, and you will suck in a more uncomfortable way, with the hand inverted or twisted around". If the patient accepts the suggestion they will become aware of the habit and it will become less pleasurable.

Massed practice involves continuous repetition of the habit until it is extinguished – a form of aversion therapy. You might suggest that the patient imagines biting their nails until their fingers are sore and bleeding. An ideomotor signal can be established, and the patient is directed to signal when they can no longer imagine themselves doing it. This may take some time, and if necessary some suggestions of encouragement and reassurance can be given to help the process along.

Milton Erickson used novel approaches to prescribing habits:

> *"I don't think you really like those stubby fingernails of yours either. And you have been biting them since you were four years old ... and I feel rather sorry for you, because for years you have been biting your fingernails and you have never gotten anything more out of it than a teensy, teensy little piece of fingernail; and you have never had a decent-sized piece of fingernail to chomp on – years of frustration! Now what I am going to suggest to you is this: you have ten fingers. Certainly you can spare one on which to grow a decent-sized fingernail, and after, bite it off, and have something worth chewing on. ...*
>
> *I pointed out to him that I thought it awfully unfair that he sucked only his left thumb; that his right thumb was just as nice and was entitled to just as much sucking, and I was astonished that he wasn't sucking his right thumb as well ... what happens is that as surely as Jimmy sucks both thumbs he has cut down sucking his left thumb by 50%. And what about the other fingers? (When you start dividing you start conquering.) ...*

> *(Can you imagine giving a turn to ten separate digits? Can you imagine a more laborious task in the world?)* ...
>
> Next I pointed out: *'you are over six years old now, and soon you will be a big boy of seven; and you know I have never seen a big boy that ever sucked his thumb, so you had better do all of your sucking before you are a big boy of seven.'* [22]

In a separate case description, he prescribes thumb-sucking in front of disapproving parents every evening. In due course, the child forgets to carry this out, and the habit is broken[10].

Anchoring

During hypnosis, memories that carry good, positive, pleasant feelings can be relived vividly, and these feelings anchored to the action of squeezing a finger and thumb together. You can then instruct the patient to start to put their hand to their mouth, but to activate the previously installed anchor just before it touches. Advise the patient that eventually there will be no inclination to begin the habit as it is no longer serving any purpose.

Aversion

Used on its own, aversion therapy is not often effective in the long term, but it may be helpful with some patients as a part of their therapy. In effect a *negative* anchor is created, linked to an unpleasant sensation such as a bad smell or taste, and the patient is taught to experience this as they are about to suck their thumb or bite their nails. Prior to using hypnosis, ask the patient to recall an experience, for instance a time when a smell or simply the sight of something made them nauseous. In hypnosis, invite them to re-experience this sensation, confirming this to you by an ideomotor signal. Finally, suggest that this feeling becomes linked to the commencement of the unwanted behaviour, so that every time the patient starts biting their nails or sucking their thumb, they simultaneously feel nauseous.

Imagery

Imagery can be a very powerful strategy for eliminating unwanted habits. It is important that the patient imagines that they are behaving as they want to behave. Encourage them to see how their nails will look, or to look forward to having a beautiful smile once they have stopped sucking their thumb. The more vivid, intense and specific the imagery and the more the patient can repeat the process, the more effective and successful it will be.

Sometimes, particularly with children, an effective strategy is for the patient to imagine someone else, such as their favourite footballer or a television character, in all the situations and circumstances where the habit is occurring (see Chapter 31). Often patients find it easier to imagine their heroes overcoming problem behaviour, and can obtain useful information and strategies from this exercise that will serve ultimately to break their habit.

Case history: Carol – reframing to eradicate thumb-sucking

The patient

Carol was aged twelve and had sucked her thumb since she was born. Her parents had tried various ways to stop this habit, including painting the thumb with bitter substances and vindaloo curry powder, bribery and threats, and none had any lasting success.

Carol's upper anterior teeth were displaced labially and there was evidence of some deformation of the anterior maxilla. She was becoming much more self-conscious about her appearance and the behaviour itself, but felt powerless to stop.

Treatment

After discussion about hypnosis, the "coin drop" induction (see Chapter 31) was used, followed by further deepening suggestions.

An ideomotor response was established (see Chapter 14) and the part responsible for the behaviour was thanked. Like most patients, Carol was happy to accept the concept of "parts" and she had commented earlier that *"it is as if there is a part of me that makes me suck my thumb".*

The part responsible was asked if it would like to "grow up" and become even more useful, and following a positive response the creative part of Carol's mind was asked to provide some alternative ways for the original part to continue fulfilling the positive intention, but in a more acceptable manner. The part that used to suck her thumb agreed to use these alternatives.

Next, an ecology check was carried out, to ensure that there was no objection to the changes, and this was followed by future pacing, whereby Carol was asked to imagine, as vividly as possible, seeing, hearing and feeling how it would be without this habit. It was suggested that she could admire her lovely even teeth and feel really pleased that she, and the original part in particular, were much more "grown up". Further suggestions for ego-strengthening were given, and Carol was complimented on how well she had done.

Outcome

As this young lady was a regular dental patient, further visits confirmed that the habit had been eradicated, and orthodontic treatment was later carried out to correct her occlusion.

30

Smoking Cessation

All psychological methods towards smoking cessation are successful to a certain extent[23, 24] but none have been shown to be completely effective. A recent Cochrane review concluded that hypnosis was as yet unproven as an anti-smoking intervention[25]. The main reason for this is that there is insufficient strong evidence (from randomised controlled clinical trials) to show that hypnosis is superior to other interventions. However, a recent review concludes that hypnosis should be considered a "possibly efficacious" treatment for smoking cessation[26]. As with other interventions for habit cessation, hypnosis for smoking cessation can be a valuable addition to our toolbox. This section will outline some useful interventions to consider.

General considerations

As always, establishing rapport together with non-judgemental empathy is essential. As smoking becomes more socially unacceptable, you must not appear condemning or condescending and must emphasise that you know how difficult it is to throw off the addiction without help.

The patient must be motivated to stop, in other words it must be *their* choice, not a response to pressure from others. The timing of the attempt to stop may be important. Concurrent high-stress situations (divorce, moving house, illness, etc.) may predispose to failure, so it may be wise to postpone the attempt.

History and treatment planning

A full history of the smoking habit will help to tailor the intervention for the particular patient.

History of the habit

- **Why do they want to stop?**
  Health, health of others, finances, smell, tooth-staining, hygiene and social acceptance may all be important.

- **Why did they start?**
  Modelling and peer pressure are often given as reasons.
  What are the particular individual aspects of their habit?

- **How many cigarettes (cigars or pipes) do they smoke?**

- **How long have they smoked?**

- **When do they smoke?**
  After meals, with alcohol, etc.

- **What does smoking do for them?**
  Stress relief, relaxation, weight control.

- **Have they tried to stop before?**
  What helped? What led to restart of the habit?

Weakening the addiction

Strategies aimed at weakening the habit can be suggested before formal hypnotic treatment. Smokers often smoke *automatically* without conscious awareness, so if this process is disrupted the habit may be weakened[27].

Altering habitual behaviour

- Use of the other hand or different finger positions when smoking.
- Change smoking routines: smoke only outside the house, cut out the coffee break or keep cigarettes out of sight or inaccessible.
- Buy only ten at a time.
- Change the brand each time a pack is bought.
- Change the supplier: go to a different shop each time.
- Gradually reduce the amount of nicotine ingested; cut down the number of cigarettes smoked, or the number of puffs taken on each cigarette.

Hypnotic procedures

This section will outline some techniques that may be used for smoking cessation. It is not intended to be exhaustive, as many regimes are available and outlined in the literature. However, this author (GT) has found these effective when used over two hypnotic sessions.

First session

Appropriate induction and deepening procedure should be followed by ego-strengthening. It is important to introduce this at an early stage as smokers may be lacking in self-confidence and self-belief.

"Each time you follow your instructions you feel more and more pleasure, more proud of your growing ability to succeed, even more determined to set yourself free."

It may also be necessary to alter the patient's attitude, suggesting that they now think in terms of "I can" or "I will", rather than "I hope I can" or "I don't think I can".

Use direct suggestions to emphasise all the benefits of being a non-smoker.

Studies have shown that individually tailored suggestions are more readily accepted than standardised suggestions[28]:

"Imagine yourself, Steve and Laura, comfortably settled in your new house, noticing how clean and fresh the curtains, walls and furniture look, and how pleasant the whole house smells ..."

"See yourself running so much more freely, smoothly, and feel how much more easily you are breathing, taking in all that wonderful fresh air ..."

The health risks can also be emphasised, once again relating to the individual patient. An apt metaphor here is the story of the person falling from a thirty-storey building, who while passing the twentieth floor says, "So far, so good!"

As smokers have illusions about the benefits of smoking, it is essential to dispel these. It is crucial to stress again and again that the *only real effect of smoking is to feed the addiction*. It can be likened to a parasite that compels the host to continue to poison itself with no real gain for the host.

Teach self-hypnosis at the first visit. This will promote relaxation and stress relief, maintain motivation, reinforce the therapy and foster the patient's self-image as a non-smoker.

Use imagery in helping the smoker to attain a new self-image as a non-smoker. One technique is negative forward pacing converted to positive forward pacing.

> *"Imagine yourself in one month's time as a smoker. Notice what you look like, smell like, how you sound, and especially how you feel. Imagine how other people feel about you, and what you think about yourself.*
>
> *Now take all the discomfort and all the harmful effects and imagine that it's six months later. Once again, look at yourself ... see the colour of your skin ... the stained teeth ... feel how your lungs are having to work that much harder to get enough air ... hear yourself coughing or wheezing after some exercise ... smell your clothes ... your rooms at home. Imagine others noticing this gradual deterioration.*
>
> *Now imagine it's five years later, and you have punished yourself and others for five more years. See, hear, smell and feel the effects on your body ... the coughing ... the teeth that are missing or loose ... the smell and taste from the increasingly unhealthy gums ... and all the other misery that tobacco has inflicted on your life.*
>
> *Now imagine that it is ten years later and if you can experience the consequences of your habit as fully as possible, and ask if you like what you see ... and how you feel ... imagine how your friends and family feel about you.*
>
> *But now, stop and breathe a sigh of relief, because it isn't ten years later. There is still time to avoid this fate. Imagine yourself in one month's time as a non-smoker. Notice what you look like ... smell like ... how you sound ... and especially how you feel. Imagine how other people feel about you ... how you feel about yourself.*
>
> *Next, imagine that it is six months later. See how you look healthier ...*
>
> *your breath is fresher and your mouth feels healthier. Notice how other people react to this improvement ... how it has benefited them.*
>
> *Now, as you imagine yourself ten years later ... when smoking is just a distant memory ... almost as if you had never smoked. See how you look ... feel how much healthier you are ... be aware of all the benefits that breaking that terrible habit has brought your friends, family and yourself. Enjoy feeling really good ... really pleased with your achievement and your sense of self-control. So, bring back all those feelings of success and self-control with you, and look forward to enjoying all those benefits, with a renewed determination to achieve them."*

Anchoring will give an association between feelings of confidence, power and being in control and being a non-smoker in response to a cue that the patient can trigger when required. Suitable triggers are to bring the thumb and finger together or to make a clenched fist (see Chapter 16).

At the end of the session, summarise the main points and stress the benefits of becoming a non-smoker and the strength of the patient's resources.

Second session

Firstly it is important to discuss how the patient feels they have progressed since the first visit. Have they changed their habit in any way? Have they practised self-hypnosis? Have they stopped smoking? Any issues must be addressed before continuing.

An important concern may be withdrawal symptoms, and you can assure the patient that these are normal and that they are transient. Withdrawal symptoms may include: cravings; respiratory tract effects (cough, dry mouth, soreness and ulceration); increased appetite; constipation and diarrhoea; sleep disruption; dizziness; mood swings and irritability.

Use self-hypnosis and anchoring to reduce the psychological effects of withdrawal. Other concerns can be reframed as positive effects of the body adjusting to life without nicotine. Instruct the patient to say, "Great, the habit is dying, soon I will be free!"

After induction of hypnosis, reinforce the fundamental suggestions made in the first session. These might include the reasons for stopping and the choice the patient made to stop. Extra imagery may be suggested where appropriate.

For example, you can ask the patient to imagine as vividly as possible a display case. Inside, sitting on velvet cushion, is an ordinary cigarette. At the front of that display case is a price tag for £20,000 (the lifetime cost to the average patient of continuing to smoke).

Stories can be added, again bearing in mind the preference of each patient.

Cancer detection

> *"Wouldn't it be wonderful if someone invented a way of predicting exactly which cigarette would start the malignant changes? So for instance they could say to you, 'The thirteenth cigarette from now will start a cancer in your lungs.' If this were possible, everyone would stop smoking before it was too late, instead of thinking 'it might not happen to me.'"*

Like flu

> *"If it were possible to have an injection that made it impossible to smoke again, but it caused unpleasant flu-like symptoms for a week or more, I think everyone would think that a small price to pay for being liberated from such a terrible addiction."*
>
> [This story helps to prepare the patient for any withdrawal effects.]

Pet food

> *"Supposing you went to buy some food for your dog, and every tin or packet of dog food had a large sign saying: 'WARNING! THIS PRODUCT COULD SERIOUSLY DAMAGE YOUR DOG'S HEALTH!' Would you seriously consider buying any? Surely you deserve to treat your own body with at least as much respect as you would a dog."*

Old friend

"Change is always stressful. Just before your appointment today I happened to come across an old photograph of myself with a friend called Dave. As boys, we were inseparable; we went to the same school, played football together and often went out with our girlfriends together. Then we went into the sixth form together, and things began to change. It soon became obvious that we were going in different directions, I intended to go on to university, Dave was just interested in having a good time. I realised that if I did what Dave wanted and kept up our close friendship, I risked missing out on what I really wanted. So, although we had had some great times, and we had some wonderful memories and nothing could take those away, I realised that the friendship could no longer go on as before. Now, one part of me missed that, and it was not easy at times, but when I look back I am so very pleased that I made the right decision, and although I can remember all the good times we had, I have absolutely no regrets

New car

"Most people find making changes uncomfortable. I remember exchanging my car last year for a newer, faster and more luxurious model. The thing was, I had driven my old car for a long time, and I was very comfortable and familiar with it. The first few times that I drove the new car, it all felt different, the controls were in a different position, the steering wheel was different, and it just felt awkward and harder to drive. I found myself thinking that maybe I should have kept the old car. However, it did not take long before I became used to all the controls and the way the car handled, and it was very obvious that it was definitely far superior. Now I would not dream of going back to the old car. It was definitely a wise decision."

Friend or enemy

"When you lose someone that you really care for, quite naturally you are upset. You miss their presence in your life, you find yourself thinking of them, remembering the things you did together, and you feel very sad. But when someone that has been nothing but trouble to you leaves your life, you are so glad, it is such a relief. Deep down you realise that tobacco has never really been your friend: a true friend would never try to harm you as tobacco does. In reality, tobacco has always been an enemy."

Reframing is another technique to be used on this second session.

Finally: end the session with positive, ego-strengthening suggestions stressing the gains of being a non-smoker and emphasising their use of self-hypnosis. Contact should be maintained as long as the ex-smoker needs it.

Dealing with lapses

It is inevitable that some patients will lapse, and return to their smoking habit. It is sometimes difficult to achieve just the right balance between a positive attitude and acknowledgment of the difficulties, and it is up to your discretion where the emphasis should lie for each patient. The ideal is to give every expectation of success but not to leave the patient thinking that one slip is irreversible. If this were to happen, the patient might resume their old patterns of smoking because they think that the treatment has been a failure. Therefore, it is essential to reframe any slip by emphasising that *a lapse is not a relapse*. It can help to suggest that the lapse is a sign of the strength of the addiction, rather than the weakness of that person.

An excellent analogy is that of learning to walk. We make numerous attempts before we manage to walk, and if we had the "this is no good, I'll never get the hang of it" attitude, we would all be crawling about in our old age. You should be supportive and encouraging, and where necessary help to increase the patient's motivation and confidence.

Advise the patient to restrict their intake of alcohol and caffeine as both can increase the risk of lapses. Some patients may find this difficult and may require further support in order to ensure success.

Lapses can also signify that other issues have not been dealt with, and further exploratory work may be necessary before the patient can cope with such a major change in their life.

Occasionally, the motivation of the patient can change. For instance, if one of their prime reasons for stopping was to save money, and they then found a much more highly paid job, won the lottery or received an inheritance, they might decide to continue smoking. Other major changes such as divorce or bereavement may occur, and these too could undermine their motivation and concentration, so that patients may find their reasons for stopping are no longer as important to them.

Case history: Muriel – smoking cessation

The patient
> Muriel was a regular dental patient, aged thirty-eight, who sought help in stopping smoking. She was well aware of the general health risks but found it difficult to relate these risks to herself. She also had periodontal disease, which was responding reasonably well to treatment. The knowledge that smoking was detrimental to the periodontal condition was a major factor in her decision to stop smoking. (It is interesting to note that quite often patients who are relatively unaffected by the risk of malignancy become very alarmed when informed that smoking may cause the loss of their teeth.)

History of smoking
> Muriel, like many other people, had started to smoke in her teens, as all her friends

and her family smoked. She had smoked for nearly twenty years, on average ten cigarettes a day. During this time she had stopped two or three times, the longest period without smoking being several months.

She admitted that for most of the time she did not really enjoy smoking, and often smoked "out of habit", but felt that when stressed, anxious or feeling run down she really needed cigarettes. On these occasions she would have "binges", where she would smoke much more than usual, and this sometimes happened when she was out drinking alcohol. She also felt that smoking helped her to keep her weight under control.

Treatment

The various considerations outlined previously in the text were then agreed, following which Muriel reiterated her wish to become a non-smoker.

Eye-roll induction was followed by progressive relaxation, a positive anchor was established and ego-strengthening suggestions were given. Muriel was then taught self-hypnosis and urged to use it daily, and the many benefits that this would provide were stressed. After ensuring her confidence in following these instructions and using self-hypnosis, a further appointment was arranged for two weeks' time.

At the next visit she reported that she had complied with all the changes, apart from occasionally smoking more than she had hoped, always when drinking and distracted.

Hypnosis was induced and I gave Muriel several of the previously mentioned analogies, following this by the reframing procedure. During future pacing, emphasis was placed on her vividly imagining herself out socialising and drinking without any need to smoke.

I also gave suggestions to help limit any weight increase, and strongly advised her to continue self-hypnosis as a way of dealing with stressful times in her life. This was coupled with ensuring that she was well aware that smoking had no real benefits, and preparing her for any withdrawal effects that may arise.

Outcome

Muriel attended four months later for a dental examination and reported that she had not smoked at all, although there had been times when she had found it difficult. At her next appointment six months later she was finding things much easier, and really felt that she would never smoke again.

References

1. Nicotine Addiction in Britain. A Report of the Royal College of Physicians Tobacco Advisory Group, 2000.

2. Oakley DA. Emptying the habit: A case of trichotillomania. Contemporary Hypnosis 1998;15(2):109–17.

3. Bandler R, Grinder J. Reframing; Neuro-Linguistic Programming and the Transformation of Meaning. Moab, UT: Real People Press, 1982.

4. Manfredini D, Landi N, Romagnoli M, Bosco M. Psychic and occlusal factors in bruxers. Aust Dent J 2004;49(2):84–9.

5. Monaco A, Ciammella NM, Marci MC, Pirro R, Giannoni M. The anxiety in bruxer child. A case-control study. Minerva Stomatologica 2002;51(6):247–50.

6. Golan HP. Temporomandibular joint disease treated with hypnosis. Am J Clin Hypn 1989;31(4):269–74.

7. Goldberg G. The psychological, physiological and hypnotic approach to bruxism in the treatment of periodontal disease. Journal of the American Society of Psychosomatic Dentistry & Medicine 1973;20(3):75–91.

8. LaCrosse MB. Understanding change: five-year follow-up of brief hypnotic treatment of chronic bruxism. Am J Clin Hypn 1994;36(4):276–81.

9. Clarke JH, Reynolds PJ. Suggestive hypnotherapy for nocturnal bruxism: a pilot study. Am J Clin Hypn 1991;33:248–53.

10. Erickson MH. The nature of hypnosis and suggestion. New York: Irvington, 1980.

11. Gow M. Hypnosis in the treatment of bruxism. In: Joint Conference BSMDH, BSECH, BSMDH (mets and south), BSMDH (Scotland), RSM(hypnosis and psychosomatic medicine section): Glasgow, 2005.

12. Heap M, Aravind KK. Hartland's Medical and Dental Hypnosis. 4th Ed. London: Churchill Livingstone, 2002.

13. Macedo CR, Machado MA, Silva AB, Prado GF. Occlusal splints for treatiing sleep bruxism (tooth grinding) (protocol). The Cochrane Database of Systematic Reviews 2005(Issue 4).

14. Macedo CR, Machado MA, Silva AB, Prado GF. Pharmacotherapy for sleep bruxism (protocol). The Cochrane Database of Systematic Reviews 2006(Issue 1).

15. Silber KP, Haynes CE. Treating nailbiting: a comparative analysis of mild aversion and competing response therapies. Behav Res Ther 1992;30(1):15–22.

16. Twohig MP, Woods DW, Marcks BA, Teng EJ. Evaluating the efficacy of habit reversal: comparison with a placebo control. J Clin Psychiat 2003;64(1):40–8.

17. Allen KW. Chronic nailbiting: a controlled comparison of competing response and mild aversion treatments. Behav Res Ther 1996;34(3):269–72.

18. Whitewood G. Hypnotic intervention in the breaking of a thumb-sucking habit. Australian Journal of Clinical Hypnotherapy and Hypnosis 1997; Mar. 18(1)1–4.

19. Ritzman TA. Nail-biting explained. Medical Hypnoanalysis Journal 1988; Jun. 3(2):48–51.

20. Tilton P. Hypnotic treatment of a child with thumb-sucking, enuresis and encopresis. Am J Clin Hypn 1980; Apr. 22(4):238–40.

21. Wagstaff GF, Royce C. Hypnosis and the treatment of nail-biting: A preliminary trial. Contemporary Hypnosis 1994;11(1):9–13.

22. Hammond DC. Handbook of Hypnotic Suggestions and Metaphors. New York: WW Norton, 1990.

23. Law M, Tang JL. An analysis of the effectiveness of interventions intended to help people stop smoking. Arch Intern Med 1995;155(18):1933–41.

24. Covino NA, Bottari M. Hypnosis, behavioral theory, and smoking cessation. Journal of Dental Education 2001;65(4).

25. Abbot NC, Stead LF, White AR, Barnes J. Hypnotherapy for smoking cessation. The Cochrane Database of Systematic Reviews 1998(Issue 2).

26. Green JP, Lynn SJ. Hypnosis and suggestion-based approaches to smoking cessation: An examination of the evidence. Int J Clin Exp Hyp 2000; Apr. 48(2):195–224.

27. Ibbotson G, Williamson A. Smoke Free and No Buts! Carmarthen: Crown House Publishing, 1998.

28. Viswesvaran C, Schmidt F. A meta-analytic comparison of the effectiveness of smoking cessation methods. J Appl Psychol 1992;77:554–61.

31

Hypnosis with Children

The child you will see as a dental patient is often the product of a background in which dentistry has a poor press. Even a caring parent may have told them that the dentist "won't hurt", thereby introducing the concept of pain. With children, possibly even more than with adults, all forms of negative suggestions must be minimised, and this particularly applies to the language that you and your staff use. Appreciate too that hypnosis is not a panacea. There will be children with whom, for a variety of reasons, it is virtually impossible to establish rapport. In some cases the immediate necessity may be for emergency extractions, and this may require a general anaesthetic. However, provided you can engage the interest of the child even to a limited extent at your first contact, it should be possible to develop rapport and to move forward on subsequent visits.

It has been proposed that when you treat a child "you treat at least three people: the child, the parent, and that child as an adult". Certainly many dentally anxious patients will relate their anxiety to an episode with a "cold, unfriendly, uncaring dentist" (see Case history: Wendy, Chapter 22).

Hypnosis can be an extremely valuable aid to dentistry with children and studies indicate that, in general, children make good hypnotic subjects. Most authorities agree that hypnotic susceptibility increases in children, being at its peak between nine and thirteen, and then gradually declines throughout life[1]. Hypnotic susceptibility is often further enhanced if children are encouraged to use their imagination in stories and play[1]. However, although children have been said to be more hypnotisable than adults with a peak at pre-adolescence, things may not be as simple as that. For example, the child's attention span may be much shorter than that of an adult and in many cases a high degree of skill is needed in order to establish rapport.

Hypnosis with a child differs from its use with adults for a number of reasons. For the young child in particular there are generally few, if any, preconceptions of hypnosis and so little explanation is necessary. The presenting problem is usually fairly clear-cut and normally there is no secondary gain involved. Quite often your major challenge will be in dealing with the parent–child relationship.

Differences between children and adults

Although, given trust and understanding, most children will accept hypnosis readily, the induction process will differ from that used with the adult patient. You will rarely use suggestions of eye-closure or relaxation, particularly when working with younger children.

Their natural curiosity and energy, and lack of cultural awareness of the expected role of the hypnotic subject, mean that children in hypnosis will behave differently from adults. This can be disconcerting if you and your surgery staff are not expecting it. The child will often appear to shift in and out of hypnosis, moving, talking, and with eyes sometimes closed and at other times open. Indeed often the child will not appear to be in the state we recognise as hypnosis, but despite that will remain deeply involved in their fantasy world. Hypnosis gives a format to relationship and sometimes can even be treated as "playing a game" with the child. Your main aim therefore is to get the child so involved in the process that they are using their vivid imagination to maximum effect.

The surgery ambience, however comfortable you may feel it to be, is likely to appear strange, alien and hostile to the young child. You and your staff might also seem huge and intimidating. Paying attention to the ambience of the surgery and welcoming the child from a seated position may help to overcome this initial barrier. It is also important that you direct remarks and questions at the child rather than talking to his parent about him over his head in the "third person invisible": "... *and how long has he been having this toothache?*" It is, however, important not to usurp the parent's role and therefore it might seem sensible to cast yourself as a favourite auntie or uncle rather than as a parental figure. In this context touch can be a valuable facilitator, particularly with the younger child, and it is imperative that this is explained to the parent and that their approval is obtained.

Right from the beginning your greeting and conversation with the child must be "user-friendly" to the child. (An actual case shown on BBC TV some years ago depicted an anaesthetist saying to a four-year-old "I'm just going to give you an intravenous anaesthetic for the operation. It'll just be a little injection and it won't hurt a bit.")

However keen the parents may be that their child has hypnosis for his dental treatment, the essential factor is that the child himself is motivated and interested. Parents will need a brief explanation of hypnosis, what it involves and what it can achieve. The child, on the other hand, will generally need little or no explanation other than that you are going to show them how they can have a good time when they have their teeth done.

Parental presence

Should a parent remain in the surgery while their child is having hypnosis? Our response to this is that as long as the parent behaves themselves they are welcome. However, there are conditions:

1) Is the child happy for the parent to stay? Does the child express a *need* for the parent to stay? Or does the child want the parent to leave? (The needs and views of the child are paramount.)
2) Will the parent accept that the relationship is between the dentist and the child and there must be no interruptions or other intervention, however well-meaning, from the parent?
3) Will the parent stand or sit quietly and out of mutual eye contact with the child?

Usually these conditions are acceptable and the whole procedure is uncomplicated. Sometimes the child may feel insecure and will initially want to have their parent around. Here you can use the *well-behaved* parent as a partner and as the child becomes more comfortable and secure in your presence you might ask the parent to gradually take a more passive role, eventually leaving the surgery.

The more anxious parent may be reluctant to stay in the surgery because of their own fears about dentistry. Here a useful strategy might be for a member of your staff, having warned the parent to be silent, quietly to invite them back when their child is happily having their treatment, while keeping out of the child's line of vision. This approach can do much to dispel anxieties the parent might have about the child, hypnosis and even their own dental treatment.

The child's world

The trust and rapport – the use of the child's language and involvement in that child's world – are the crucial factors behind using hypnosis successfully with children. In order to build this rapport it is important to find out as much as possible about their likes and dislikes, hobbies and interests, favourite TV programme and character, favourite computer games and so on.

If the procedure is likely to involve TV-watching, it is important that this is placed in the right context. Maybe the child has a favourite room and chair or bit of floor from which they watch TV, and maybe they are alone or with their best friend or a parent. However, it is important that you give the child the freedom to choose this. A statement such as " ... sitting on your mother's knee in your sitting room ..." may cause discordance, whereas "... in your favourite place ... maybe on your own ... maybe with someone you really like ..." will give the child that choice.

Obviously the choice of words and phrases you will employ in speaking with children differ from adult language and, in general, the younger the child the simpler the words and style you will use. Quite often, it may be simpler to begin talking to the child without any explanation, simply introducing the process as telling them a story. Formal deepening is normally not needed as the storytelling itself will accomplish this. Remember that the child will probably not understand words such as "imagination" and "relaxation", and so you might use alternatives such as "comfy", and "tell me if you can see this picture even when your eyes are closed" or "just like watching telly". Remember too that most children, particularly the younger ones, will have no concept of hypnosis, and so words normally associated with sleep, such as "dreamy … drowsy … sleepy" can be very acceptable.

Working with children it becomes even more important to use their (preferred) name, more often than with adults. This will give the child a sense of importance, will increase rapport and will also tend to focus their attention on what you are saying and its applicability to themselves. Remember that children tend to have a short attention span, so ideas should be presented in very small chunks.

Compliance will also be increased by the use of permissive-sounding phrases rather than orders. For example, compare the effect of "… close your eyes and you can see pictures behind your eyes …" with "… I wonder if, when you close your eyes, you can see pictures behind them … I bet you can …". By making instructions sound almost like a challenging game, you are more likely to raise the child's interest, so phrases such as "… I bet you can't …" and "… do you know that … ?" will gain the child's cooperation.

"Tell, show, do"?

A number of authorities propose the "tell, show, do" procedure as a useful form of desensitisation for the nervous child. But this is reinforcing the dental scene, however gently, to the child. In using hypnosis one is attempting in effect to "take the child away" from the dental scene. As you will find from our examples, it is important when using hypnosis to forewarn the child of certain possible sensations, but more often the "tell and show" can be used *after* the dental treatment and hypnosis, when it can act as a very powerful form of ego-strengthening.

> "… gosh, you have done SO well … do you know what you have just done? … would you like me to show you? …"

Never lie to a child; they will find you out and all chance of rapport will be lost. This becomes an issue when the child asks either "will you be giving me a needle?" or "was that an injection?". If the question is asked after the local has been given, this can be used as ego-strengthening as described above, but the question asked before the procedure is more problematic. In this instance the "tell, show, do" technique is sometimes beneficial provided the "tell" is focused on the positive aspects, such as the use of "magic" cream and the comfort of a good anaesthetic.

Uses of hypnosis

As with adults, hypnosis is a facilitator for any and all dental procedures with children and is particularly effective in the circumstances listed below. For practical purposes the age limit will probably be around six years, although younger children are also sometimes suitable.

Uses of hypnosis in dentistry for children

- Management of fear and anxiety
- Pain control in conservation and extractions
- Impression-taking
- Fissure sealing
- Where the child needs to be still for a long time (e.g. orthodontic procedures)
- As an adjunct to inhalation sedation
- As part of the induction of general anaesthesia
- Habit elimination (thumb-sucking, nail-biting)

Table 31.1 **Synopsis of induction techniques** (adapted from K. Olnes[1])

Age	Strategy
0-2 years	Tactile stimulation, stroking, patting, etc. Kinesthetic stimulation, rocking, moving an arm back and forth Auditory stimulation, music or other soothing sounds Visual stimulation, mobiles, etc. Dolls and stuffed animals
2-4 years	Blowing bubbles Storytelling Favourite activities Puppets
4-6 years	Breathing Favourite place Guided fantasy, e.g. flower garden, beach, football game, etc. Storytelling Coin-watching Television fantasy Bouncing ball or ball in a bucket Videos Biofeedback Finger-lowering
7-11 years	As above Video games, real and imagined Riding a bike Arm-lowering Favourite music Hands moving together
12-18 years	Most adult methods, especially: Fantasy methods, e.g. video and computer games Music, real and imagined

Some general notes on techniques with children

Although it is our intention within this section to describe the use of hypnosis with dental patients from approximately six years old upwards, we will preface it with a few words suggesting techniques for use with the younger child. Here the well-behaved parent can be a valuable silent ally, and provided you can get the full attention of the child there is no reason why they should not sit on their parent's knee.

Although children under six may enter a trance-like state, hypnosis for dental treatment is not realistic unless the operator has specialist skills. Even when the child is over the age of six you must use your judgement regarding their maturity and likely cooperation to decide whether or not you feel hypnosis will be the strategy of choice. In all of the cases described below, we will assume that rapport has been developed with the child and that the parent has given the requisite approval and permission for the procedure.

Some induction methods for the very young child

In the days of the cord-driven slow handpiece, the late George Fairfull Smith[2] used a beautiful technique in which he would attach pieces of cotton wool to the drive cord and gently get the little child to concentrate on watching "... the wee foxy-woxy chasing the little bunny rabbit". Lulled by Fairfull-Smith's gentle Scottish burr, the child would enter a trance state in which the dental work would be tenderly carried out.

A modern-day alternative is to have available a number of dolls, toy animals and puppets with which you can enact the child's problem in metaphorical form, generally bringing into the story sleepiness, dreaminess and the solution to the problem (see the discussion of metaphors later in this chapter).

The slightly older child

Smiley thumb levitation
This is a simple technique that incorporates involvement, arm levitation and eye closure, and can be used with dental patients from approximately six years old upwards.

Begin by drawing the familiar smiley face on the child's thumb nail. You might also start by asking the child what colour they would like you to use, and what name they are going to call the face. Show the child how to hold his arm out straight and slightly raised with the thumb nail clearly visible, and ask them to stare at the smiley face as hard as they can.

> *"... so Suzie ... I wonder if you can keep staring at Billy as hard as you can ... and the funniest thing is that the harder you stare, Suzie ... it's as if Billy really wants to look at your face ... and ever so slowly, Suzie, he's going to float up ... right up to your face ... and then it becomes magic ... 'cos when Billy just touches your face ... your eyes close ... and you'll feel so dreamy ... drowsy ... and sleepy ... and it's just like you're in your special place ... and you're watching your very best thing on telly ... and, Suzie ... now Billy can just flop down and go to sleep and you can just watch ..."*
> [here describe the programme that the child has previously told you of]

Smiley thumb heaviness

Begin as above, but rather than suggesting arm elevation suggest:

> *"... and now, Suzie ... the harder you stare at Billy ... do you know what's going to happen ... Billy is going to get so-o-o heavy ... heavier and heavier ... and so tired ... and sleepier and sleepier ... and I wonder how long it'll take, Suzie, before Billy is so heavy and tired and sleepy ... that soon, Suzie ... he's going to be fast asleep ..."*
> [take hand and rest it comfortably and continue with TV dream as above]

Coin drop

This method, in addition to the game-playing and involvement of the child, also carries the promise of a minimal bribe. The idea is that you give the child a (low-denomination) coin and ask them to hold it with their arm raised and at arm's length between thumb and forefinger.

> *"... Debbie ... I wonder if you can stare really hard at that coin ... really hard, Debbie ... and as you do, I think your arm is going to get heavier and heavier ... really so heavy, Debbie ... and tired ... and soon it'll feel so very heavy and tired that that coin will just drop on its own ...* [here it is sensible to be ready to catch the coin as it falls, to avoid noise]
>
> *... and it doesn't matter, Debbie 'cos we'll keep it safe for you for later ... and as it drops you'll be so dreamy and drowsy and sleepy that ..."*
> [take hand and rest it comfortably and continue with TV dream as above]

Informal dissociation by TV imagery

This technique will utilise the child's natural ability to daydream, and this will be coupled with your status and the status and responsibility you have given to the child by treating them as a person.

Rapport can be enhanced by a brief discussion with the child to determine their interests, siblings, pets, TV viewing habits and so on. Wording and language should obviously be appropriate to the child's age, and tone should be friendly and conversational, giving the child the feeling that this is a very personal and important meeting.

Eye closure might be suggested, but at this stage is not important (see below).

Case history: Simon – a TV dream

The patient
Simon was a particularly bright and imaginative boy aged six. His mother, Judy, had previously suffered from severe dental phobia and I had used hypnosis with her, after which she had become an excellent and happy dental patient. Simon had probably been influenced by his mother's earlier dental anxieties and was quite obviously terrified about the two deciduous tooth fillings he now needed. Judy prepared Simon well by telling him how gentle and kind I was, and how with me he could have a "special dream about Popeye" (his favourite television character). Simon asked if it was going to be hypnosis and Judy told him that it was. At that stage Simon said he wanted his mother to stay and they both agreed that she would sit quietly in a corner of the surgery.

Treatment plan
My plan was to use hypnosis informally with Simon, particularly as his mother had prepared him to the extent even of the content of his dream. Our rapport was good and I felt we could use his powerful imagination to create sufficient dissociation for me to carry out the two fillings without local anaesthetic.

Procedure
[beginning in slow conversational mode and moving into quieter, slower, dreamy hypnotic tones]

"... Now, Simon ... you know when you want to see pictures sort of in your head ... do you do it best when your eyes are shut or open?" (Simon said it was best with his eyes closed)

"... so why don't you just close your eyes ... and I know that you like Popeye ... so here's what you can do ... do you have a best place when you watch telly, Simon? [Simon nodded] ... I bet you can see that now ... your best place ... just how you like it ... .and there's Popeye on the telly ... he's so strong and so funny and maybe he's got a tin of spinach ... and maybe Olive Oyl's there as well ... that very, very, very thin lady ... and Bluto ... isn't he huge ... I wonder what they're doing ... I bet you can make up the story, Simon ... maybe you can even be in the story ...

[here, using "vague exactness", a story involving a tin of spinach and Popeye's success was described]

... and now it's nearly finished ... and I bet Popeye's won again 'cos he always wins ... and now it's all finished and you can open your eyes again ... and I'm here and mum is here and you have been amazing Simon ... and guess what ... we've made those teeth all better for you and all the time you've just been having a lovely dream watching telly ..."

During this time (about 10 minutes) I prepared cavities with a slow-speed drill in both lower Es and restored them in amalgam. Simon occasionally moved a little and opened his eyes on a couple of occasions, but was obviously comfortable and happy, to the extent that I didn't sense a need even to explain to him what I was doing or to prepare him for the different sounds or sensations, and he made no response to them.

An amusing sequel
Simon from then on was a model patient and apparently had few anxieties regarding dentistry. However, there was an amusing sequel about two years after this episode when his mother told me that he had confided in her, telling her, *"It can't have been hypnosis 'cos although I told the dentist I was dreaming about Popeye I was really dreaming about Tom and Jerry!"*

Another informal technique

You will have noted that in the previous example dental work was barely mentioned. In the following case the child is given suggestions preparing her for each subsequent stage of her experience of dentistry.

Observe that the language and imagery and verbal delivery employed are hypnotic. Note, too, the important step of warmly congratulating Pam on achieving each target. This will help to strengthen rapport, encourage further goal-setting and act as a powerful form of ego-strengthening.

Case history: Pam – reframing the treatment

The patient
Pam was a very anxious six-year-old girl with pain in an upper deciduous molar needing urgent treatment. She'd never attended a dental practice before and her mother was not a patient.

Treatment plan

After gaining the parent's consent, it was planned that I would relieve Pam's pain without distressing her, and at the same time begin to build up her trust and confidence, using an informal storytelling approach.

Procedure

I began by chatting about her school, her friends, TV programmes and so on before explaining that some nasty little "bugs" had eaten their way into her tooth, and this is why it was hurting. I asked her if she would like me to gently chase these bugs away, then clean up after them, give it a good wash and fill in the hole that the bugs had made so they could not get back in. After Pam had agreed, the explanation continued, quietly and rhythmically, as she began to be more and more involved in the story.

She was allowed to see and smell the "magic jelly" (flavoured topical anaesthetic) that would start to send that part of her mouth to sleep. This was then gently placed next to the upper left first deciduous molar, suggesting that the bugs were starting to get sleepy.

Next, when the surface of her gum was "asleep" (this was tested by carefully touching that area) I would squirt some "magic water" at that place so that everything went to sleep in and around the painful tooth. I explained that she would feel something, and gently pinched her hand telling her that would be just like it would feel near her tooth:

"Some little girls say it feels like a tickle, others say it is like a squeeze, I wonder what you will say it felt like?"

I told her that although she did not have to, the magic worked better if she closed her eyes, and when she did so, the injection was given very slowly while asking her to think about all the bugs going to sleep, just like Sleeping Beauty. When the injection was given, Pam was praised lavishly and congratulated on helping the magic to work so well.

Then, she was shown a probe and the point was carefully pressed onto her hand. When she said that her mouth was feeling "bigger" the probe was pressed against the gum at the side of her tooth. When the girl confirmed that she could not feel it like she could when it touched her hand, the praise was repeated and she was told that all the bugs would be fast asleep.

Next, she was shown the slow handpiece, which I described as a "tickling machine".

I started the handpiece and slowly let it play over my arm, before allowing it to run over her finger. When she felt this, she shivered and giggled, and I told her that when the bugs were tickled they all came out of the hole in her tooth. By now the little girl was so interested in what was happening she was not aware of the previous pain.

The tooth was gently made caries free, with a continuous commentary on how all the bugs were running away. She was shown some of the caries and she was amazed to see the "sleeping bugs". After this, I praised her again for being so good. Then I explained that because the bugs were so dirty (she had seen the brown slush previously) the hole needed to be washed out and vacuumed, like her mother did at home, so everything was nice and clean. I showed Pam the water syringe and aspirator tube. She was a little apprehensive at first, mainly because of the noise, but after she had felt it on her hand, and after a "practice", where the tube was held next to the tooth very briefly, she allowed the cavity to be flushed. Once again, Pam was highly praised.

The next step was to start filling in the hole, firstly with some "special paint", and some calcium hydroxide was placed. Then it was time for some more magic. She was shown some glass ionomer cement and was told that by shining a "magic light" I would make the cream turn very hard, sealing up the hole. The filling was then cured.

Finally, Pam was told enthusiastically how well she had done. Both the girl and her mother were very pleased.

Outcome

Over the next few weeks a similar routine was followed to restore her other carious teeth, and Pam now attends regularly without anxiety.

The "ball in bucket" game
(with acknowledgement to Don Ibrahim)

In this technique you will introduce the child to your suggested imagery and incorporate "automatic movement", arm levitation and a useful bribe.

Case history: Sam – ball in bucket and arm levitation

The patient
Sam was a very active six-year-old who needed a small filling in a deciduous tooth, but possibly did not even *know* how to sit still. It seemed sensible to use an induction method that would take advantage of his restlessness.

Strategy.
"*... and Sam, we are now going to play a little game. You'd like that, wouldn't you? ... and with this game you'll see lots of pictures of some lovely things ... and you'll able to see them even with your eyes closed ... doesn't that sound great, Sam ... are you ready ... super ... so now I'd like you to close at your eyes ... that's lovely ... and I wonder if you can see a picture behind your eyes, Sam ... and the picture is a bucket of a water ... just like the sort of bucket you might have if you go to the seaside ... can you see that? ... and what colour is the bucket? ... blue? ...*

[it is important to get a positive response here to indicate that the child has created an image] ... *that sounds really lovely, Sam ... and can you see that there's water nearly to the top of the bucket? ... good ... and on top of that water there's a ball floating ... can you see that? ... and what colour is that ball? ... red ... so there's a red ball floating on the water in that blue bucket ... and now we're going to play our game, Sam ... I'll just take your hand and I'm going to put it on top of the ball ...*

[I lifted his left hand and positioned it as if on top of a ball about 30 cm (12 inches) above the armrest, keeping my hand above and gently holding his wrist] *... and I wonder if you can push the ball down into the water ...*
... and what happens? ... yes, isn't it funny how it floats back up [I moved Sam's hand slowly up and down, establishing automatic movement] *... and down again ... and up ... and down again ... and up ...*
... I wonder if you can just carry on doing that on at your own ... [I let him continue the motion] *... up ... down ... up ... down ... and now a funny thing will happen ... because that ball is going to turn into balloon ... a beautiful big balloon ... and do you know what? ... it's going to float up higher and higher and your hand will float up with it, Sam ... and when your hand floats up to your face the balloon can just float away, and it doesn't matter because we've got another balloon here for you later ...*

And now, Sam ... you can just let your hand brush against your face ... and when it does you will start to feel really dreamy and drowsy and sleepy ... and you can just let your hand drop back down and ...
[continued as in earlier examples]

Dissociative techniques

A number of imaginative techniques particularly applicable to the older child have been described by Karen Olness[1].

Switching a sensation on and off
Using language appropriate to the child's age, suggest in hypnosis that the child visualises some form of switch, for example a light switch, push-button or lever, and then practises turning that switch on and off. Propose to the child that the switch turns on and off the connections from the various parts of the body to the brain, so that they cannot feel a certain area, such as the part of the mouth that needs attention.

Computer analogy
The computer now plays a large part in the lives of many children, and its potential as a hypnotic metaphor is boundless. Build on the suggestion that the child is sitting before their computer, gazing at the screen, and let them set up their own programs to deal with their present difficulty. This may involve wiping the current behaviour program, rebooting the computer and setting an alternative, or placing a current document in the "recycling bin".

The vast array of computer games available to children and their ability to manipulate them also opens up many opportunities for hypnotic imagination and involvement. These opportunities can be used to wipe out any obstacles to change or to achieve any goals that may be required.

Detachment
Ask the child to imagine that a part of them does not belong to them; as if it is detached from them, or is artificial, so that any sensation there cannot be felt. This can be enhanced by getting the child to imagine a mask or a doll/toy animal facing them and transferring all sensation to the equivalent area on the imagined toy. Be sure to build in the sense of security that at the end of the session they will be whole again.

Displacement
Ask the child to "imagine that all the feelings are going into your little finger on this hand, then, after it has all gone into that finger, you may want to let it just float away".

Alteration of cognitive variables
Some children find it difficult to be distracted or to dissociate. An alternative is to ask the child to give a detailed description of their discomfort, and you can then gradually give suggestions that change their perception for the better. Depending on the age and inclination of the child, responses can be given either verbally or by an ideomotor response.

The questioning might then be as follows:

"Has it got a colour?"
"Or has it got a shape?"
"What size is it?"
"Is it rough, or is it smooth?"
"Does it make a noise?"
"Does it have a smell?"
"What colour/size/shape/texture/sound/smell would it have to be to feel better? I wonder if you can start to change it [to a more desirable characteristic]"

Glove analgesia

A variation of the imagery as used for adults (see Chapter 25) can be effective for an appreciable number of children. You might say, for example:

> *"I wonder if you've ever been playing in the snow and maybe you lost a glove, or your gloves got ever so cold and wet ... and your hand was so cold that you could move your fingers, and just couldn't feel anything at all..."* [on receiving a positive response this can be extended into transferring the resultant numbness to the area of the dental work]

Stories and metaphors with children

> *"Once upon a time the famous physicist Albert Einstein was confronted by an overly concerned woman who sought advice on how to raise her small son to become a successful scientist. In particular she wanted to know what kinds of books she should read to her son. 'Fairy tales', Einstein responded without hesitation. 'Fine, but what else should I read to him after that?' the mother asked. 'More fairy tales', replied the great scientist, and he waved his pipe like a wizard pronouncing a happy end to a long adventure."* (Breaking the Magic Spell[3])

Storytelling is a hypnotic technique. It can produce the distinctive narrowing of focus of attention, altered sensation and time distortion that characterise hypnosis.

The power of stories and metaphors lies in their ability to be understood on several levels.

- *Superficially:* as entertainment or distraction.
- *Deeper:* as a reminder of other story times, such as being at home feeling contented at bedtime.
- *Deeper still:* as a representation of a part of the child's life or experience. The story may suggest solutions, or at least give a role model for the child to emulate.

Any parent who has read to their children must be aware of a child's ability to become totally immersed in a story and the almost ritualistic role the story can take on in that child's life. Children will have a favourite bedtime story and in a short space of time, even for a normally excitable child, this can become an anchor to peacefulness, settling down and sleep. Sometimes one might be reading a child a much-loved story while the child is apparently totally engrossed in some other activity and the child will instantly snap into awareness if a single word is omitted or altered. We are surrounded by such evidence of the child's ability to dissociate; to become absorbed in fantasy at the expense of reality. Much of children's game-playing involves the acting out of make-believe characters who to the child's mind can assume reality. Sometimes the barrier that for most adults separates fantasy from reality seems barely to exist in the world of the child.

Stories and game-playing therefore present you with a remarkably effective route to utilising these qualities within hypnosis in dentistry.

> *"For a story truly to hold the child's attention, it must entertain him and arouse his curiosity. But to enrich his life, it must stimulate his imagination; help him to develop his intellect and to clarify his emotions; be attuned to his anxieties and aspirations; give full recognition to his difficulties, while at the same time suggesting solutions to the problems which perturb him. In short, it must at one and the same time relate to all aspects of his personality – and this without ever belittling but, on the contrary, giving full credence to the seriousness of the child's predicaments, while simultaneously promoting confidence in himself and in his future."*
> Bettleheim[4]

Ingredients of a therapeutic metaphor

For a metaphor to be used successfully it should ideally contain certain key elements. Here we will present a real case study followed by a deconstruction in order to point out these elements.

Case history: George –
a Liverpool Football Club supporter

> *The patient*
> George was an eight-year-old boy who came along crying with pain from a very carious upper deciduous molar. He was extremely distressed and nervous, and not in the mood even to let someone look at the tooth. I noticed that he had a Liverpool football bag and so I started to talk about football, especially the Liverpool team.

Treatment plan

My intention was to use a dissociative technique. I would tell George a story centred around the football team, using the "another person" metaphor and gradually integrating George into this character and into the story. I planned to inject local anaesthetic and to extract the carious tooth

"Do you remember when Steven Gerrard had very bad toothache just before the last Champions League match? [George gave a hesitant nod] ... *well, it was really painful, but he knew that unless he went to the dentist and let him sort it out, he would not be able to play well in the big match. Now, how do you think Steven Gerrard was when he went to the dentist? Can you imagine him going in to the dentist, and listening to what the dentist had to say? Although Steven Gerrard knows lots and lots about football, he also knew that dentists know lots and lots about making toothache better, and because he trusted the dentist, he knew that he had to do whatever the dentist said to make that toothache go away, so he would be ready for the big match.*

Now, shall we do the same things that Steven Gerrard and the dentist did?
[George nodded again]

Great! ... the dentist told him that he would make the tooth and the gum around it go to sleep. First he would rub some special ointment on his gum, just like the ointment that they use when footballers get injured in a game. So, shall we do that?
[George nodded]

Next, the dentist told him that he would squirt some liquid at the place where the gum was starting to go to sleep, and do you know what Steven Gerrard did? He closed his eyes so that he could imagine that he was playing in the big game. And guess what, if you close your eyes, you will be able to imagine that you are playing in that game with Steven Gerrard, and all the other Liverpool players! So, let me know when you can imagine yourself walking out onto the pitch ...
[after a few moments George nodded again]

Now I'm going to squirt that liquid and you will probably feel something ... Steven Gerrard said it felt a bit tingly [the injection was given slowly and evenly, at the same time as further suggestions about the game were being made] ... *can you hear how loud the fans are cheering? And can you hear some of the songs?*
[and so on]

That was brilliant – just like Steven Gerrard! So, you can let yourself get right on with the game, has it kicked off yet? [once again, George nodded) *Good, now you will have*

concentrate on the game so that you play at your very best, and of course, when you play in a big game like that, you get pushed and pulled about a lot ... [I pushed his arm, and tugged at his shirt while saying this] *... and you can get pushed on your body, your legs, your arms and even on your face, around your mouth ...* [all these statements were accompanied by some pushing and pulling] *... but you can handle that, playing for Liverpool, you know that you are the best! And you know that you always get pushed and pulled, it's all part of the game, but it does not stop you from scoring goals, does it? And I bet if you play really well now, even though the other team are trying very hard to stop you, you can score!* [the tooth was quickly extracted, without any pause in the dialogue] *... even when they try and foul you, they can't stop you from scoring, and the fans are chanting, they are chanting your name!*

So, when the game is over, you can open your eyes, you have done ever so well, just like Steven Gerrard! I can't wait for you to tell me the score!"

Outcome

After a short time, the boy opened his eyes. He seemed a little bemused, but with myself and his mother and the dental nurse all telling him how well he had done, he was able to leave the surgery calmly, marvelling at the extracted tooth that we had given him.

Analysis of this case

1) The story must interest the child and must meet the child at his level without imposing the view of the therapist. An effective way of doing this is to interweave elements of the child's particular interests, for instance their favourite animals or TV programmes, within the story.

"... Do you remember when Steven Gerrard had very bad toothache just before the last Champions League match? ... well, it was really painful, but he knew that unless he went to the dentist and let him sort it out, he would not be able to play well in the big match ..."

2) The story must represent the child's problem accurately enough for them to identify with the characters and events portrayed. The significant events and characters of the child's real situation must be present in the metaphor, preserving the relationships and emotions, but not the context.

"... Although Steven Gerrard knows lots and lots about football, he also knew that dentists know lots and lots about making toothache better, and because he trusted the dentist, he knew that he had to do whatever the dentist said to make that toothache go away, so he would be ready for the big match ..."

3) The goals represented within the metaphor must be realistically within the reach of the child.

"... and because he trusted the dentist, he knew that he had to do whatever the dentist said to make that toothache go away, so he would be ready for the big match. Now, shall we do the same things that Steven Gerrard and the dentist did?"

4) The emotional content of the metaphor should be strong and must mirror the child's experience

"... and of course, when you play in a big game like that, you get pushed and pulled about a lot ... and you can get pushed on your body, your legs, your arms and even on your face, around your mouth ... but you can handle that, playing for Liverpool, you know that you are the best!"

5) The metaphor must show a resolution to the problem, and indicate how the child can achieve this.

"And you know that you always get pushed and pulled, it's all part of the game, but it does not stop you from scoring goals, does it? And I bet if you play really well now, even though the other team are trying very hard to stop you, you can score!"

6) There must be a celebration at the end to show the child that there is a reason to change and to acknowledge their effort and achievement.

"... even when they try and foul you, they can't stop you from scoring, and the fans are chanting, they are chanting your name!

So, when the game is over, you can open your eyes, you have done ever so well, just like Steven Gerrard! I can't wait for you to tell me the score!"

Other person metaphors

A few moments spent in identifying the child's interests, pets, icons and anti-heroes will pay rich dividends, and with practice you will find that you are able to build simple stories such as this. It can be incorporated into a story about "another child": "I once saw a pretty little girl just like you ..."

A further way of using this technique is to compose a story in which the child's hero succeeds in conquering a problem analogous to the one that the child has.

For the young child the doll or animal can be used as the metaphor, and you might talk to the animal in much the way you would to the child, at the same time possibly making it slightly more dramatic or comical.

Fairy tales and cartoons

One of the simplest ways of constructing metaphors is to take as a "template" characters and situations with which the child is already acquainted. The fables of Aesop and the stories of the Brothers Grimm and Hans Christian Andersen offer a wealth of material, and it is not difficult to modify the story and even to include the child as one of the characters, confronting problems and attaining success and glory at the end.

In a similar vein many children are fixated on children's TV cartoons and characters, and this may be exploited in a similar way.

It is important that you adhere to the key elements referred to above and essential that the story ends in triumph. After all, the child will have heard enough stories giving the negative side of dentistry.

"I think a job like this requires
The services of Mr Myers."
I shouted, "Not the dentist! No!
Oh mum why don't you have a go?"
I begged her twice, I begged her thrice
But grown-ups never take advice.
She said, "A dentist's very strong.
He pulls things out the whole day long."
She drove me quickly into town,
And then they turned me upside down
Upon the awful dentist's chair,
While two strong nurses held me there.
Enter the dreaded Mr Myers
Waving a massive pair of pliers ...

He started pulling one by one
And yelling "My, oh my, what fun!"
I shouted, "Help!" I shouted "Ow!"
He said, "It's nearly over now.
For heaven's sake, don't squirm about!
Here goes! The last ones coming out!" ...

From *"The Porcupine"* by Roald Dahl[6]

Remember: all explanations are stories – make yours good ones!

32

Hypnosis as an Adjunct to Sedation

The way that we communicate with patients, both verbally and by our body language, has a profound effect on their response. In addition, a person's emotional state will affect their suggestibility. This is particularly important when we look at hypnotic suggestion as an adjunct to the range of conscious sedation techniques used in dentistry.

For some years now, the use of sedation in dentistry has been advocated as an alternative to general anaesthesia (GA). Concerns about the safety of GA have meant that its use is now restricted to the hospital setting, and as a result dentists have sought alternatives.

In 1990, the influential "Poswillo Report"[7] began this process and the Department of Health document "A Conscious Decision"[8] set out the agenda for a change in the approach and use of sedation and GA. Slightly different definitions of conscious sedation are given by the two reports (Table 32.1).

Table 32.1 **Comparison of the "Poswillo Report" and "A Conscious Decision".**

"Poswillo" 1990[7], p.4	**"A Conscious Decision" 2000[8], p.8**
"A carefully controlled technique in which a single intravenous drug or a combination of oxygen and nitrous oxide, is *used to reinforce hypnotic suggestion and reassurance* in a way which allows dental treatment to be performed with minimal physiological and psychological stress, but which allows verbal contact with the patient to be maintained at all times. The technique must carry a margin of safety wide enough to render unintended loss of consciousness unlikely." [*emphasis added*]	"A technique in which the use of a drug or drugs produces a state of depression of the central nervous system enabling treatment to be carried out, but during which verbal contact with the patient is maintained throughout the period of sedation. The drugs and techniques used to provide conscious sedation for dental treatment should carry a margin of safety wide enough to render loss of consciousness unlikely."

Poswillo criticised the existing definitions of sedation on the grounds that they failed to recognise the essential basic element of hypnotic suggestion and reassurance, and emphasised central nervous system depression rather than mood alteration.

As yet, the ideal sedation agent does not exist. Currently the commonly used methods are: inhalation sedation (IHS, nitrous oxide/oxygen sedation, relative analgesia); oral sedation and intravenous (IV) sedation (usually midazolam).

This chapter will demonstrate how these techniques can be enhanced by their combination with hypnosis.

Inhalation sedation agents

The main agent used for inhalation sedation is nitrous oxide/oxygen mixture (N_2O/O_2).

Table 32.2 **Properties of an ideal sedation agent compared with N_2O/O_2 sedation and IV sedation with midazolam**

Ideal property	N_2O/O_2 sedation	IV sedation with midazolam
Allows treatment	Relatively weak agent, large variation of response	Powerful agent, effective for very anxious or phobic individuals[9]. Not effective in 100% of cases.
Safety	Safe for the patient. Very few side effects, no adverse effects on liver, kidney, brain, cardiovascular or respiratory system[10]. High levels of oxygen used during the technique make it the treatment of choice for patients with certain medical conditions[11].	Not suitable for children or adults with medical conditions, because of respiratory depression[9]. Careful clinical and electro-mechanical monitoring is required[9, 10].
Margin of safety between sedation and general anaesthesia	Large margin of safety in an adequately oxygenated patient because of high minimum alveolar concentration (MAC) (over 80) – theoretically impossible to produce anaesthesia when used alone with adequate oxygen[9].	Reasonably large margin of safety between sedation and anaesthesia, but over-sedation possible – wide variation in response, difficult to establish endpoint of sedation[12].
Simple, pleasant painless method of administration	No injections required – method of choice in needle phobia. Technique operator-sensitive – use of semi-hypnotic suggestion necessary for success[9].	Venepuncture necessary. Difficult for dentist, unpleasant for patient, especially if needle phobic[10].

Table 32.2 (continued)

Ideal property	N₂O/O₂ sedation	IV sedation with midazolam
Rapid onset	Onset of action is more rapid than oral, rectal and intramuscular (IM) injection. Approximately equal to intravenous (IV) injection[10]. Due to low blood gas partition coefficient and relative insolubility[9].	Most rapid onset of all technques, arm-brain circulation time is 20-25 seconds[10]. Full clinical effect takes several minutes.
Predictable action and duration	Only currently available technique having variable duration of action under control of the clinician. Depth of sedation variable, according to demands of the situation and the patient[10]. Action fairly predictable, at least in children, as an alternative to general anaesthesia (83.4% success rate in 3-16 years age group)[13].	More predictable action than N₂O/O₂ but disinhibition may occur[9]. Ineffective in reducing anxiety for some patients[14]. Duration of action predictable – 40 minutes (approx.) working time[9].
Rapid recovery	Recovery rapid, usually complete after 3-5 minutes breathing 100% oxygen. Only technique allowing adult patients to be unaccompanied[10].	Recovery shorter than oral or IM[10]. Patient usually fit for discharge <2 hours after procedure[9]. Recovery not complete – escort needed[10]. Reversal possible by Flumazenil (only for emergency use).
Rapid metabolism and excretion	N₂O minimally metabolised, elimination from the lungs rapid[9].	Metabolised in liver, excreted by kidney – elimination half-life 1.9 hours, +/- 0.9.
Analgesia	Good analgesic (20% N₂O/O₂ equivalent to 10-15 mg morphine[10].	No analgesic properties.
Compatibility with other drugs	Good.	Interactions with many drugs possible.
Low incidence of side effects	Yes.	No information collected on morbidity associated with sedation[8].

IHS sedation has a number of advantages summarised in Table 32.2.

Despite its advantages, N_2O/O_2 is not an ideal sedation agent. The equipment is expensive and bulky and the technique requires considerable cooperation from the patient. In addition, because of the lack of potency of the agent, some patients fail to respond to the technique[10]. Some dental procedures (e.g. surgical treatment in the anterior part of the mouth) are difficult to carry out[15]. The major disadvantage is danger to dental personnel, N_2O traces in the atmosphere having been implicated in a range of haematological, neurological, reproductive, hepatic and renal problems[9, 10]. There is also potential for abuse.

Intravenous sedatives

Midazolam has replaced other benzodiazepines as the drug of choice for intravenous sedation because of its shorter elimination and recovery time (compared with diazepam)[9]. The major advantage over IHS is the more powerful sedative action. Good levels of amnesia are achieved, which may be related to patient satisfaction with the technique[14], although amnesia can also be a drawback leading to problems on the second visit and difficulty when educating the patient to accept normal dentistry[9].

The use of hypnosis in combination with sedation

Sedation should be reserved for those highly anxious patients who cannot tolerate dental treatment any other way. The pharmacology of sedation agents, while highly effective in many cases, is often insufficient to reduce anxiety about dental treatment, and so what you do before the treatment session may be just as important as what you do during treatment. Rapport-building and the avoidance of negative suggestions is even more important in highly anxious individuals.

It has been proposed that dental phobics may be more suggestible than the population in general, and this high suggestibility may contribute towards their phobia mediated by negative suggestions given inadvertently by dentists or acquired from societal discourse[16].

Inhalation sedation

The words we use and the way in which we use them are an integral part of all dental sedation techniques. Studies have shown that the successful use of inhalation sedation depends on the technique of the operator, who must keep up a steady stream of reassuring "semi-hypnotic" patter throughout the procedure[17]. In addition, the inhalation of nitrous oxide and oxygen may facilitate the acceptance of hypnotic suggestions when compared with a placebo administration of oxygen[18]. Knowledge of how to formulate and deliver hypnotically styled suggestions would be a valuable tool to anyone intending to use this technique.

The actions of nitrous oxide have been shown to be influenced by the type and amount of information given, even without using hypnosis. Dworkin and his co-workers showed that when people were given more information about how nitrous oxide worked to control pain, their experience of pain was considerably reduced[19]. More interestingly, in a separate experiment they increased pain perception with nitrous oxide/oxygen mixtures by telling the participants that nitrous oxide could increase awareness of sensation[20].

Integrating hypnosis into IHS technique

Hypnosis can be introduced formally or used informally as an integral part of IHS sedation. If a patient has had a previously unsatisfactory experience, the formal use of hypnosis may be necessary to convince them that you are doing something special. Shaw and Welbury[21] describe using hypnotic imagery in a group of children previously unable to accept dental extractions with IHS and LA. The addition of hypnotic imagery enabled treatment to be carried out in the majority of these cases.

Although IHS is often thought of as a technique mainly for children, it can be used very successfully with anxious adult patients. Children may be more imaginative than adults, although they do not always understand what is meant by "relaxation". Words such as "sleepy", "floppy", "dreamy" or "like a rag doll" may be more successful. When using the technique for either adults or children, do not be afraid to use "childlike" language. "Happy air" is a commonly used name for IHS and is acceptable for both adults and children.

Hypnotic induction (whether formal or informal) can begin at the introductory stage of the IHS technique when the patient is breathing just oxygen. Because you are asking them to concentrate on breathing slowly and deeply in and out through the nose, techniques linked to breathing, for instance, imagining breathing in calmness and "coloured air", and breathing out any anxiety as they let the breath go, work well. Progressive muscular relaxation linked to the "out breath" is also useful.

For some individuals you may find that the hypnotic induction and relaxation thus produced is enough to enable treatment to be carried out at this stage, without the nitrous oxide. Don't remove the nose-piece, because if the patient believes that they *need* the sedation this may ruin their relaxation. However, always let them know at the end that they have succeeded by their own efforts.

If the patient requires it, nitrous oxide should then be titrated as normal until the patient is sufficiently relaxed. Suitable deepening techniques should be linked to the actions of the sedation, and suggestions of warmth, tingling sensations and comfort are readily accepted. IHS produces feelings of dissociation that can also be utilised as deepening techniques. Ask the patient what sort of sensations they are experiencing and use these to deepen their relaxation and comfort. One patient described to me that she felt as though she was floating in a warm sea. Such a statement is a gift and should immediately be built up using all sensory modalities. For others, the use of "special place" imagery uses the dissociation to allow the patient to fantasise while the dental procedure is carried out and to return when it is complete. It is not necessary to know where the special place is, although it is sometimes advantageous to agree on one before hand so that descriptions can be more specific.

Once treatment is nearing completion, post-hypnotic suggestion should be used, remembering that the aim is ultimately to wean the patient away from IHS. Post-hypnotic suggestions that the next session will be even more relaxing and that relaxation will happen automatically on sitting in the dental chair are appropriate. Finally, as the patient breathes the necessary 2–5 minutes of pure oxygen at the end of the session, ego-strengthening suggestions appropriate to the success achieved should be given.

IHS without the machine?

One patient (treated by C.P.) who had experienced IHS and liked it presented at the practice where we had no IHS facilities. Using hypnosis she was able to recreate the pleasant experience, from the feeling of the mask on her nose, the smell of the nitrous oxide and the relaxation, enabling treatment to proceed easily. Once anxious patients have experienced dental treatment in a relaxed manner, with or without sedation, they can recreate the experience, with the help of hypnosis and sympathetic treatment.

Suggested script for use with IHS for adults:

Progressive muscular relaxation

"As you breathe the happy air ... you may notice the changes that happen in your body ... you can feel warm and comfortable ... and as you breathe out your body tends to settle down in the chair and you can feel more relaxed ... First, concentrate on the muscles of your face ... as you breathe just let them relax. And now spread that relaxation down ... down to the muscles of your neck ... and your shoulders ... just let all those muscles relax, completely relaxed ... as you breathe, let all the tension drain away, as if the happy air is taking all the tension away. That's right. And now spread that relaxation down through your arms, your hands ... right down to the very tips of your fingers ... Notice how the tips of your fingers can feel so relaxed, warm and comfortable ... notice any tingling sensations at the very tips of your fingers and how comfortable that can feel. Next, spread that relaxation down through your chest and your back ... through your chest muscles, and your back muscles, as you breathe, just let them relax. And now ... through the stomach, and the hips ... let that warmth and relaxation spread down ... comfortably and easily into your legs. Down ... through your legs ... your knees ... your calves ... into your feet ... right down to the very tips of your toes ... until the tips of your toes can feel just as warm, tingly and relaxed as the rest of your body. That's great. And you know ... when you relax like this ... everything that we do can feel so comfortable and you can feel completely calm, completely controlled, comfortable and relaxed."

Now special place imagery can be introduced:

Special place imagery

"When you relax like this, your mind can choose for you a special place, a place where you can feel ... calm, controlled, comfortable and completely relaxed. It may be a real place that you have visited in the past, ... or it may be completely imaginary. Just allow your mind to come up with a place like that right now. A special place ... where you can feel calm controlled comfortable and completely relaxed. When you have found your special place, just let me know with a nod of your head. OK, now allow yourself to be in that special place ... see all the sights you can see, the colours and shapes, maybe people ... Hear the sounds you can hear ... Even smell any smells there may be. Let yourself really be there in your special place, and feel those good feelings of calmness, comfort and relaxation. You can stay in your special place for as long as you want to right now and enjoy those feelings ... just allow all the stresses and strains of the work day to disappear ... And each and every time you need to de-stress you can make your way back to your special place ... and you ... don't need to do anything, just enjoy being in your special place ..." [the patient can stay in the special place until the dental treatment is complete]

Ego-strengthening and arousal (while the patient is breathing 100% oxygen)

"In a short while our time together today will be over ... Just use the last few minutes to enjoy that feeling of complete relaxation ... Take a few minutes to feel really good about what you have achieved today ... You have had your dental work done ... and been so relaxed, so comfortable, so calm ... And that can make you so proud.

You can know that the next time you come here ... you can achieve this relaxation, much more quickly ... much more easily ... In fact, just as soon as you sit down on the chair, you will start to relax ... When you put the nose 'bobble' on for the happy air, you will relax more and more, so that we can work to make your mouth more and more healthy.

Just allow yourself to feel really proud of your achievements today ... Then when I count to three, you can drift back to the here and now, bringing back with you everything you want to remember and everything you need to remember ... And enough relaxation and mental calmness to allow yourself to enjoy the rest of the day. Ready ... one ... two ... three."

Combining hypnosis with intravenous sedation

Intravenous sedation has become more accepted recently as an alternative to general anaesthesia for patients who are highly anxious and for patients undergoing unpleasant procedures such as wisdom tooth removal. One problem that has been identified with the technique is that patients may become overly dependent upon it, and it is more difficult to wean a patient off the use of IV sedation than IHS. Hypnosis may have a place in helping to achieve this and to facilitate the use of IV sedation in patients who are initially so anxious that GA may seem the only choice.

Intravenous sedation is a powerful technique that relies on true pharmacological sedation rather than the so-called psycho-sedation represented by IHS. This has been taken by some to mean that behavioural techniques are not important while using it, and while it is true that adequate sedation can be achieved simply by the correct use of the drug (usually midazolam), it is possible to use hypnosis to enhance the success of treatment. This has been shown to be effective for several groups of patients: medically compromised[22], drug-dependent[23] and pediatric patients[24]. In these case series, the authors either reduced the amount of sedative agent required to produce adequate sedation, or treated patients who were previously untreatable under sedation.

A further series of cases showed significantly less stress (measured by heart rate increase), a reduction in sedative drugs and a shorter recovery time for the group having wisdom teeth removed with a combination of hypnosis and IV sedation with midazolam and fentanyl, compared with patients who received IV sedation alone[25].

One problem with the use of IV sedation is that significant amnesia usually covers the entire procedure, so the patient does not have the opportunity to learn from their experience. Indeed, they may return for a second visit insisting that last time they were anaesthetised, or that the sedation must have been better, because they have no memory of the event. Most patients, however, can remember everything prior to the sedation taking effect, so hypnosis to alleviate their anxiety can usefully precede the sedation.

Although no studies have yet been published in this area, the use of hypnotic techniques to reduce anxiety should ultimately enable a patient to accept treatment without sedation.

Needle-phobic patients present a barrier to the use of IV sedation, so hypnosis can be used to treat the needle phobia to enable the patient to accept venepuncture. The pain of venepuncture and cannulation is also perceived as a barrier to IV sedation techniques, so techniques such as glove analgesia can be used to combat this. Careful choice of methods for production of glove analgesia is necessary as techniques suggesting that the hand becomes cold and numb may cause difficulties in finding a vein. It is preferable to use suggestions incorporating hand-warming aimed at increasing peripheral blood flow.

Conclusions

Sedation techniques are increasingly used in hospital and general dental practice as an alternative to GA, both to alleviate patient anxiety and for unpleasant procedures such as wisdom tooth extraction. Hypnosis can be integrated into both inhalation and intravenous sedation techniques to improve patient acceptance of treatment and to help anxious patients ultimately accept treatment without the use of chemical sedation.

References and suggested reading

1. Olness K, Kohen D. Hypnosis and Hypnotherapy with Children. 3rd Ed. New York: The Guilford Press, 1996.
2. Fairfull Smith GW. The modulation of fear, anxiety and pain with hypnosis. SAAD Digest 1976;3(4):76–9.
3. Zipes JD. Breaking the Magic Spell: Radical Theories of Folk and Fairy Tales. London: Heinemann, 1979.
4. Bettleheim B. The Uses of Enchantment: The Meaning and Importance of Fairy Tales. New York: Knopf, distributed by Random House, 1976.
5. Gordon DC. Therapeutic Metaphors : Helping Others Through the Looking Glass. Cupertino, CA: Meta Publications, 1978.
6. Dahl R. Dirty Beasts. London: Jonathan Cape, 1983.
7. Poswillo DE. General anaesthesia, Sedation and Resuscitation in Dentistry: Report of an Expert Working Party. London: HMSO, 1990.
8. A Conscious Decision. A Review of the Use of General Anaesthesia and Conscious Sedation in Primary Dental Care: Report by a group chaired by the Chief Medical Officer and Chief Dental Officer: Department of Health, 2000.
9. Girdler NM, Hill CM. Sedation in Dentistry. Oxford: Wright, 1998.
10. Malamed SF. Sedation: A Guide to Patient Management. St Louis, MO: Mosby, 1995.
11. Robb ND. Sedation in practice Part 4: The use of sedation for the medically compromised patient. Dental Update 1977;24:54–9.
12. Richards A, Griffith M, Scully C. Wide variation in patient response to midazolam sedation for outpatient oral surgery. Oral Surg Oral Med O 1993;76;4:408–11.
13. Blain KM, Hill FJ. The use of inhalation sedation and local anaesthesia as an alternative to general anaesthesia for dental extractions in children. Brit Dent J 1998;184; 12:608–11.
14. Ellis S. Response to intravenous midazolam sedation in general dental practice. Brit Dent J 1996;180;11:417–20.
15. Robb ND. Sedation in dentistry Part 1: Assessment of patients. Dental Update 1996;May:153–6.
16. Gerschman JA, Burrows GD. Dental anxiety disorders and hypnotizability. In: Mehrstedt M, Wikstrom P-O, eds. Hypnosis in Dentistry. Hypnosis International Monographs No.3. Munich: M.E.G.-Stiftung, 1997.
17. Roberts GJ. Inhalation sedation (relative analgesia) with oxygen/nitrous oxide gas mixtures Part 1: Principles. Dental Update 1990;17, 4:139–45.
18. Barber J, Donaldson D, Ramras S, Allen GD. The relationship between nitrous oxide conscious sedation and the hypnotic state. J Am Dent Assoc 1979;Oct. 99(4):624–6.
19. Dworkin S, Chen A, Shubert M, Clark D. Cognitive modification of pain: Information in combination with N-sub-2O. Pain 1984;19(4):339–51.
20. Dworkin SF, Chen ACN, Leresche L, Clark DW. Cognitive reversal of expected nitrous-oxide analgesia for acute pain. Anesth Analg 1983;62(12):1073–7.
21. Shaw AJ, Welbury RR. The use of hypnosis in a sedation clinic for dental extractions in children: report of 20 cases. ASDC J Dent Child 1996; Nov-Dec;63 (6):418–20.
22. Lu DP, Lu GP. Hypnosis and pharmacological sedation for medically compromised patients. Compend Contin Educ Dent 1996;Jan;17(1):34–6.
23. Lu DP, Lu GP, Hersh EV. Augmenting sedation with hypnosis in drug-dependent patients. Anesth Prog 1995;42(3-4):139–43.

24. Lu DP. The use of hypnosis for smooth sedation induction and reduction of postoperative violent emergencies from anesthesia in pediatric dental patients. ASDC J Dent Child 1994;May–Jun. 61(3):182-5.

25. Dyas R. Augmenting intravenous sedation with hypnosis, a controlled retrospective study. Contemporary Hypnosis 2001;18, 3:128-34.

Part 8

Appendix

Ethical Considerations and Safety Aspects

1) Do I always use the word "hypnosis"?

This question crops up at every course and workshop on which the authors have worked, and shows a genuinely expressed concern, hence its inclusion here. There may be many occasions when you use some simple informal techniques to help the patient relax and feel less anxious. Many dentists with no formal training in hypnosis will intuitively use relaxation and imaginative methods to de-stress patients.

Certainly practitioners in various other fields of professional care use virtually identical techniques under such titles as relaxation and visualisation, guided imagery, psychoprophylaxis, relaxation therapy and autogenic training. In such circumstances, even though these suggestions could be classed as hypnotic, it is not unethical to refer to them instead simply as "relaxation with imagery". Indeed, some people who may at first be opposed to the idea of hypnosis would happily accept such a form of treatment under a different nomenclature. In such situations there is no question of deceiving the patient, and if the patient were to ask afterwards "Was that hypnosis?", the similarities outlined above could be used within your explanation. Added to this might be the fact that many people will go into this trance-like state of their own accord at times when they feel sufficiently secure and comfortable. It is, however, important that unless you have specifically entered an agreement with the patient that you will use hypnosis, any hypnotic phenomena such as ideomotor signalling and hypno-analgesia should not be contemplated.

It may be helpful here to quote from "*The Nature of Hypnosis*"[1]:

(i) Hypnotic Induction

"A session of hypnosis normally begins with a 'hypnotic induction'. This usually consists of a series of suggestions that direct the subject to relax and to become absorbed in their inner experiences, such as feelings, thoughts and imagery" (page 3[1]).

(ii) General nature of hypnotherapeutic procedures

"Hypnotherapeutic approaches typically involve induction and deepening methods that usually emphasise mental and physical relaxation ...

Hypnotherapeutic procedures resemble and overlap with other therapeutic methods such as covert behaviour therapy, meditation, relaxation therapy, autogenic training and guided imagery techniques. Hence it is not uncommon for two therapists to be using very similar procedures, one calling them 'hypnosis' and the other using one of the aforementioned terms" (page 9[1]).

(iii) Training in the therapeutic application of hypnosis

"Training in hypnosis for the purposes of applying it therapeutically should, therefore, only be undertaken by individuals who already possess or are in the process of acquiring, professional qualifications and experience in understanding and treating those problems for which they intend using hypnosis" (page 13[1]).

The corollary of (i), (ii) and (iii) above is that a practitioner using "relaxation therapy" and "guided imagery" should remain cognisant of the training requirements, contra-indications and precautions regarding hypnosis described elsewhere within this Appendix.

As you develop skills and a reputation as a dentist who uses hypnosis, increasing numbers of patients will attend your practice with specific requests for hypnosis for their dental treatment. If hypnosis is directly referred to and is to be used, then it is necessary to obtain informed consent. This means that the patient must be informed what the treatment will involve and what it can and cannot do, and invited to ask questions in order to obtain as much relevant information as they may need. It should also be explained that they, the patient, will be in control and that the process therefore requires them to play an active part in it.

2) Physical contact

Dentistry inevitably involves physical contact and it is easy to take this for granted; however, it is important to get permission to touch the patient if this is intended during hypnosis. This contact may be during the induction or in setting up an anchor, but if the patient is not expecting that contact it can startle or upset them, especially if the hypnosis has been progressing for a while and they have their eyes closed.

3) Chaperone

It is strongly recommended that at all times when you are in your surgery with a patient a chaperone, normally your nurse, is present. As you develop your practice of dental hypnosis there may come times, for example in the case of extreme dental anxiety, when the patient will be so reluctant to enter the surgery that the consultation will have to be held in a "neutral" consulting room. In this setting the patient and possibly you yourself will be inhibited by the presence of a third party. A nurse or receptionist should always be close by, perhaps in an adjacent room.

In any professional relationship there is the risk of an accusation of improper behaviour, perhaps more so in hypnosis as the patient will normally have their eyes closed and within their therapy they may be fantasising, and possibly experiencing a range of powerful emotions. It should be emphasised that the essential for any therapeutic intervention is trust, and that in such a trusting relationship, particularly when the outcome is successful, the potential for harmful allegations is small, but at the same time it must not be ignored.

It may be possible to record the treatment, either by video or audio, and if this is proposed patient consent is necessary. It is also important that you reassure the patient that any records so made will be kept securely and that no third party will have access to them. Obviously, as with any dental treatment, it is essential that you record all the details of the interaction in the patient's records.

When treating children, the consent of the parent or guardian is needed before you use hypnosis in any formal way. Whether or not the adult is present will depend on the age of the child. Generally speaking younger children will tend to want someone with them, and the parent or guardian will also want to be present. Any adult who stays in the surgery with their child should be asked to remain quiet and preferably out of the direct eye-line of the child. It is important that the relationship in the surgery is between you and the child without the parent acting as an intermediary.

4) Adverse responses to hypnosis

Occasionally patients may report disagreeable after-effects following hypnosis, and this might negatively affect their feelings about having further sessions. Effects may include headaches or anxiety, confusion or disorientation. These effects may be due to a patient's faulty expectations of hypnosis, but more probably are the result of the form of induction – for example, excessive eye-roll – or from a failure on your part to "lay to rest" any sensitive trance imagery prior to alerting the patient. If such after-effects do occur it is sensible, having listened to the patient's story, to reassure them and to allay their confusion and discomfort:

> "... let's help you to deal with this ... why don't you just close your eyes and let your breath out and just let go ... and as you relax give your body and mind space and time to come gently back to normal ... so much more comfortable again ... putting away those images for the time being ... and in a few moments ... you'll start to feel ready to become alert and awake ... and you'll feel so much more comfortable in your mind and your body ... and then you'll slowly count in your mind down from five to one ... and at one open your eyes ... wide awake, refreshed, relaxed ... comfortable and alert ..."

5) Abreaction

An abreaction is an emotional release or discharge that can occur during hypnosis, when the patient recalls a painful experience. Potentially, abreaction is beneficial, allowing some desensitisation of the distressing emotions or giving the patient greater insight into their experiences.

Management of abreaction is described in Chapter 22 of this book.

Contraindications to the use of hypnosis

The Clinician

Clinicians should not work outside their own areas of training and competence.

> *"Increasingly ... there is developing a conviction that the hypnotic state or process itself poses no inherent dangers for patients but that its inexpert use may. The solution to prevent potential patient harm is to ensure that all clinicians of whatever discipline have adequate and appropriate clinical training prior to being allowed to practice"*[2], quoted in National Guidelines for the Use of Complementary Therapies in Supportive and Palliative Care[3].

The Patient

Psychiatric status: where any psychiatric condition exists that may lead to unpredictable behaviour and responses, hypnosis is contraindicated.

Emotional status: depression is often a concomitant of cancer. Effective treatment of depression in cancer patients results in better patient adjustment, reduced symptoms and reduced cost of care, and may influence disease course[4]. When using hypnosis, the lack of clinical expertise specifically in working with the depressed person may only serve to compound their problem.

Inappropriate age: the major criterion is that the patient is aware of the process and its aims. This will tend to exclude the very young (possibly below six years) and the very old (although chronological age is less relevant than overall awareness).

Precautions

> *"With ... real authorities, agreement is almost unanimous that dangers (of hypnosis) are minimal and can be avoided. In some instances there have been bad results, but they have come because of personality difficulties of the hypnotist, authoritative, coercive use of hypnosis, or lack of knowledge. Patients will protect themselves from harm when the therapist shows respect for their ability to do so"*[5].

It is helpful and usual to explain to the patient the likely process of the hypnotic intervention, to remove any doubts and fears, and to obtain the approval and consent of the patient.

Obviously the clinician should be acutely aware of the legal implications of working with a patient who is in a state of hyper-suggestibility, and who (generally) will have their eyes closed.

Abreaction, a (possibly powerful) emotional response to recalled images and feelings, may be triggered off by hypnosis. This is particularly likely where the patient is already under considerable emotional pressure. The clinician should be trained and competent in using skills to protect and work with the patient, and to re-orientate the patient following an abreaction.

Before alerting a patient, any suggestions other than those intended to be post-hypnotic should be removed. For example, if anaesthesia had been produced it is important to terminate it[5].

Post-hypnotic suggestions should be time- and situation-specific.

Alerting should be gradual, and it is important that the clinician ensures that the patient is fully alerted before concluding that session.

Practitioner training and qualifications

Training

The British Society of Medical and Dental Hypnosis (BSMDH) is a national and federal organisation that offers training in hypnosis to professionals with a conventional health-care qualification who are employed in a substantive post with the NHS. Training is at basic, intermediate and advanced levels, and members are encouraged to pursue training towards accreditation by BSMDH. The core curriculum is set at national level, and training is organised at branch level. In order to maintain consistent standards, a selection of (branch level) courses are attended annually by observers from other branches.

Society	Telephone	Website	Email
BSMDH	07000560309	www.bsmdh.com	natoffice@bsmdh.com
BSMDH (Metropolitan and South)	0208 905 4342	www.mercurysky.co.uk/bsmdh	valentinela@talk21.com
BSMDH (Scotland)	0141552 1606	www.bsmdh-scot.org.uk	mail@bsmdh-scot.org.uk
BSECH	01457 839363	www.BSECH.com	ann@williamson.co.uk
RSM	020 7290 2986	www.rsm.ac.uk/hypnosis	
Hypnosis Unit UK		www.hypnosisunituk.com	info@hypnosisunituk.com

BSMDH views hypnosis as an additional skill/tool for professionals with a conventional health-care qualification, to be used alongside their primary role (e.g. as a doctor, dentist or nurse), and within the expertise of their primary qualification. From the perspective of BSMDH, the ethics and clinical responsibility that come with working with a person in a hypnotised state are such that those practising hypnosis should already have a primary professional reason to be in a helping relationship with patients, be able to accept clinical responsibility for their actions, and have indemnity cover.

The British Society of Experimental and Clinical Hypnosis (BSECH) works closely with the BSMDH and offers some courses, but does not accredit practitioners. Although open to other professionals, membership comprises mainly psychologists who may or may not be trained in hypnosis.

Regulatory bodies

BSMDH and its branches, and BSECH are the two professional organisations in the UK whose members practise hypnosis integrated with the professional's primary (conventional) health-care role. Members are answerable to, and follow the codes of ethics, conduct, etc. of, their own (primary) professional body.

References

1. Heap M, Alden P, Brown R, Naish P, Oakley D, Wagstaff G, et al. The Nature of Hypnosis. A report prepared by a working party at the request of The Professional Affairs Board of the British Psychological Society, 2001.
2. Stanley R, Rose L, Burrows G. Professional training in the practice of hypnosis the Australian experience. Am J Clin Hypn 1998; Jul. 41(1):29–37.
3. National Guidelines for the Use of Complementary Therapies in Supportive and Palliative Care. The Prince of Wales's Foundation for Integrated Health, 2003.
4. Spiegel D. Cancer and Depression. Brit J Psychiat Suppl 1996; Jun. (30):109–16.
5. Cheek D, LeCron L. Clinical Hypnotherapy. New York: Grune & Stratton, 1968.

A leaflet explaining the use of a relaxation CD

Your relaxation CD

Take time once or twice a day to play the CD, preferably on a personal player with headphones, and make it almost like a ritual in your life. Remember that the time you spend in relaxation is YOUR time. Tell this to your family. Put a "Do Not Disturb" sign on the door. Take the phone off the hook.
Be selfish. This is YOUR time.

Relax either in bed or in a comfortable armchair. Get as comfortable as possible. Unfold your arms and uncross your legs. Gradually allow your breathing to become gentler and slower. Let the pressures ease. Each time you exhale, "let everything go" as if each time you breathe out it's like a gentle sigh of relief.
Then switch on the CD.

The first time or two you'll possibly find you're analysing what's happening. You may be a little self-conscious. You'll possibly find that your mind goes off on tangents. Don't worry! This is all absolutely normal. As with everything else, you will improve with practice, and over a short period you'll get into the habit of just going along with the suggestions on the CD.

Be assured that if anything happens during your relaxation time that demands your attention, you'll instantly be wide awake and alert and ready to deal with it. Remember: relaxation alone is a way of conserving your energy and helping you to feel fitter, stronger and happier, both mentally and physically. When once you've mastered relaxation you are ready, if you wish, to move onto further stages in managing other more specific problems and their effects on your life.

Good luck!

The following is a suggested template for the wording of a Practice Leaflet introducing patients to hypnosis:

HAPPY TEETH DENTAL PRACTICE
12, The Square,
Anytown
Phone: 022 222222
Email: Happyteeth@hotmail.com

At this Practice we often use hypnosis to help patients to deal with any worries or concerns about dentistry.

Why don't you ask the receptionist for further details, or mention it to your dentist.

We are here to help you!

****

Anne Smith BDS

Anne has a vast experience of dentistry and knows that many patients have fears and concerns about dentistry.

Because of this she has studied ways of helping people to feel more comfortable when having their dental treatment.

Anne is an Accredited member of BSMDH, the foremost organisation in the UK for training doctors and dentists in the use of hypnosis with their patients, and has used hypnosis to help a great number of patients at "Happy Teeth".

****

What is hypnosis?
Hypnosis is a natural, enjoyable and very beneficial process that helps you to use your mind to achieve more control over your thoughts, feelings and behaviour.
It feels similar to daydreaming, or the moments just before waking or going to sleep, and most people find it incredibly pleasant and very relaxing.

****
How does it work?
In hypnosis appropriate positive suggestions can have a much more powerful effect. Because of that you'll find that you can make some remarkable and often rapid changes so that you are able to have your dental treatment much more easily and comfortably.

What is self-hypnosis?

Your dentist might also teach you "self-hypnosis" so that you are able to use your new ability on your own whenever you feel the need, giving you back your sense of control.

****

Is hypnosis safe?

In hypnosis, you will not be asleep or unconscious so you will remain in control at all times. Consequently it is a safe and rewarding experience.

****

Can anyone use hypnosis?

People vary in the way that they experience hypnosis but almost everyone can use it. It is not something that is done to you, but something that comes from within yourself, with no loss of control at any time.

****

What can it be used for?

Hypnosis is used very successfully for a wide range of problems and conditions. In dentistry it is a very successful way of controlling fear and anxiety, making dental treatment much more pleasant for you.

At the Practice we use hypnosis to help people deal with many problems:

Phobias – Fears about any aspects of dental treatment.
Pain relief – Gagging and saliva control – Anxiety, stress and panic attacks
Smoking cessation
Habits such as nail-biting, thumb-sucking, tooth-grinding, together with sedation

Index